FIRST AID
for the
USMLE
STEP 2
A Student-to-Student Guide

ANGELICA GO
University of Wisconsin Medical School,
Class of 1995

MARIA TERESA CURET-SALIM
University of Wisconsin Medical School,
Class of 1995

NATHANIEL FULLERTON
University of Wisconsin Medical School,
Class of 1995

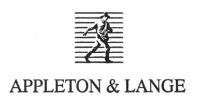

APPLETON & LANGE

Copyright © 1996 by Appleton & Lange
A Simon & Schuster Company

96 97 98 99 / 10 9 8 7 6 5 4 3 2 1

Prentice Hall International (UK) Limited, *London*
Prentice Hall of Australia Pty. Limited, *Sydney*
Prentice Hall of Canada, Inc., *Toronto*
Prentice Hall Hispanoamericana, S.A., *Mexico*
Prentice Hall of India Private Limited, *New Delhi*
Prentice Hall of Japan, Inc., *Tokyo*
Simon & Schuster Asia Pte. Ltd., *Singapore*
Editora Prentice Hall do Brasil Ltda., *Rio de Janeiro*
Prentice Hall, *Englewood Cliffs, New Jersey*

ISBN 0-8385-2591-1

9 780838 525913

90000

Acquisitions Senior Editor: John J. Dolan
Managing Editor, Development: Gregory Huth
Production Services: Rainbow Graphics, Inc.

PRINTED IN THE UNITED STATES OF AMERICA

Contents

Acknowledgments

This has been a collaborative project from the start. We gratefully acknowledge the thoughtful comments, corrections, and suggestions of the numerous medical students and faculty who have supported the authors in developing *First Aid for the USMLE Step 2.*

We also thank Vikas Bhushan, Tao Le, and Chirag Amin, the authors of *First Aid for the USMLE Step 1,* who successfully developed the first Student-to-Student guides for our publisher, Appleton & Lange, and to John Dolan, Senior Editor, and Gregory R. Huth, Managing Editor, on the project.

Finally, a very special thank you goes out to: David Jewell, Manager, Professional and Technical Books Department, University Book Store at the University of Wisconsin—Madison.

Michael Moninger, Student Academic Development, University of Wisconsin Medical School.

The Classes of 1994 and 1995 at the University of Wisconsin Medical School.

Preface

At this point in our careers, we have just finished with a year-and-a-half stint that started when we took Step I, included third-year rotations, and led to the "high pressure" (ie, vital to the Match) rotations of fourth year. With the Match looming ahead, most of us would appreciate a little help—something to make this last hurdle of our graduate medical education less stressful, a little easier. And that is what *First Aid for the USMLE Step 2* is meant to do.

In the first section, we introduce the exam. Our aim here is to make the format more familiar to you, as well as to help you organize your planning for the exam. It is our hope that knowing the "whys," the "hows," and the "whats" pertaining to the exam will help you feel more comfortable with Step 2.

The second section provides a brief review of the most vital facts you must know for the exam. Most of these topics were generated from surveys of medical students who took the Step 2 exam in the fall and spring of the last 2 years. These surveys were completed shortly after taking the exam and were designed to gather the "high-yield" topics found on Step 2. This second section is meant to aid your fact review. We believe that if you know and understand these topics, you will have the minimum needed to pass the exam.

Finally, our last section reviews the books available to use in your review for the Boards. We have evaluated these books specifically for their applicability to Step 2. We looked at the quality and accuracy of questions and explanations, readability, length, and cost. We hope to make your search for resources easier and quicker, whether you are looking for a more complete general source or specialty books to help you bone up on specific topics. We have also included a review of other books you might use during your clinical years. These textbooks and handbooks were evaluated primarily on their usefulness for rotations or for future use during residency. Some of these may also be useful for Boards review.

We hope you will find our book useful and that it will make preparing for Step 2 easier for you. We would greatly appreciate any comments, suggestions, or criticisms you might have for our book. Remember, this is the last big hurdle of medical school. Good luck!

The Authors

Abbreviations

ABG	arterial blood gas		LV	left ventricle
abx	antibiotics		LVH	left ventricular hypertrophy
AOM	acute otitis media		MMR	mumps—measles—rubella vaccine
ASD	atrial septal defect		NG	nasogastric tube
bx	biopsy		nL	normal
Ca	cancer		NTG	nitroglycerin
CBC	complete blood count		OCP	oral contraceptive pill
CK	creatine kinase		OM	otitis media
CK-MB	creatine kinase, myocardial band		OPV	oral polio vaccine
CO	cardiac output		PAOP	pulmonary arterial occlusion (wedge) pressure
CRP	C-reactive protein		PCWP	pulmonary capillary wedge pressure
CSF	cerebrospinal fluid		PDA	patent ductus arteriosus
CT	computed tomography		PE	physical exam
CVP	central venous pressure		PID	pelvic inflammatory disease
cx	culture		PMNs	polymononuclear cells
CXR	chest x-ray		PS	pulmonic stenosis
D/C	discharge or discontinue		RAD	right axis deviation
dx	diagnosis		RLQ	right lower quadrant
dz	disease		RV	right ventricle
EBV	Epstein–Barr virus		RVH	right ventricular hypertrophy
ECF	extracellular fluid		S_1	1st heart sound
EEG	electroencephalogram		S_2	2nd heart sound
ECG	electrocardiogram		SLE	systemic lupus erythematosus
ESR	sedimentation rate		SVR	systemic vascular resistance
EtOH	alcohol		sx, sxs	symptom, symptoms
F/U	follow-up		tx	therapy or treatment
GI	gastrointestinal		TM	tympanic membrane
HBIG	hepatitis B immunoglobulin		TPA	tissue plasminogen activator
HBV	hepatitis B vaccine		UA	urinalysis
HR	heart rate		ULSB	upper left sternal border
HSP	Henoch–Schönlein purpura		URI	upper respiratory infection
IM	intramuscular		U/S	ultrasound
IV	intravenous		VSD	ventricular septal defect
LAD	left axis deviation			
LLSB	lower left sternal border			

How to Contribute

Here's your opportunity to join the hundreds of faculty and student reviewers whose contributions have made *First Aid for the USMLE* student-to-student guides possible.

Please send us your suggestions for:

■ New facts, mnemonics, diagrams, or strategies
■ High-yield topics that may reappear on future Step 2 exams
■ Personal ratings and comments on review books that you have examined.

Diagrams, tables, partial entries, updates, corrections, and study hints are also welcome. Also let us know about material in this edition that you feel is low-yield and should not be included in the future.

Send entries, neatly written or typed or on disk (Microsoft Word 6.0 or earlier version or WordPerfect 5.1 for DOS) to: First Aid for the USMLE Step 2, Appleton & Lange, P.O. Box 120041, Stamford, CT 06912-0041, Attention: Contributions. Please use the contribution and survey forms on the following pages. (Attach additional pages as needed.)

You are also invited to send us your entire annotated *First Aid for the USMLE Step 2.* Contributions received by June 15, 1996, receive priority consideration for the next edition.

Note to Contributors
All entries are subject to editing and review. Please verify carefully all data and spellings. In the event that similar or identical entries are submitted, only the first entry received will be used. Include a reference to a standard textbook to help in our verification of additional medical facts. Please follow the style, punctuation, and format of this edition, if possible.

Contributor Forms

begin on page xi

Contribution Form I

For entries, mnemonics, facts,
strategies, corrections,
diagrams, etc.

Contributor Name: _____

School/Affiliation: _____

Address: _____

_____

Telephone: _____

Topic:

Fact and Description:

Notes, Diagrams, and Mnemonics:

Reference:

Return Address

_____

_____

_____

Postage
required

Attn: Contributions
First Aid for the USMLE Step 2
Appleton & Lange
107 Elm Street
P.O. Box 120041
Stamford, CT 06912–0041

Contribution Form II

For high-yield topics for
Section II Supplement

Contributor Name: _____

School/Affiliation: _____

Address: _____

_____

Telephone: _____

Please place the subject headings (eg, Pediatrics) on the first line and the high-yield topic on the following two lines.

1. Subject: _____
   Topic: _____
   _____

2. Subject: _____
   Topic: _____
   _____

3. Subject: _____
   Topic: _____
   _____

4. Subject: _____
   Topic: _____
   _____

5. Subject: _____
   Topic: _____
   _____

6. Subject: _____
   Topic: _____
   _____

7. Subject: _____
   Topic: _____
   _____

8. Subject: _____
   Topic: _____
   _____

9. Subject: _____
   Topic: _____
   _____

10. Subject: _____
    Topic: _____
    _____

Return Address

_____

_____

_____

Postage
required

Attn: Contributions
First Aid for the USMLE Step 2
Appleton & Lange
107 Elm Street
P.O. Box 120041
Stamford, CT 06912–0041

Contribution Form III

For review book ratings for
Section III

Contributor Name: _____

School/Affiliation: _____

Address: _____

_____

Telephone: _____

We welcome additional comments on review books rated in Section III as well as reviews of texts not rated in Section III.
Please fill out each review entry as completely as possible. Please do not leave "Comments" blank. Rate texts using the letter
grading scale provided on p. 84, taking into consideration other books on that subject.

1. **Title/Author:** _____

   Publisher/Series: _____ ISBN Number: _____

   Format: _____ No. of Questions: _____

   Rating: _____ **Comments:** _____

   _____

   _____

2. **Title/Author:** _____

   Publisher/Series: _____ ISBN Number: _____

   Format: _____ No. of Questions: _____

   Rating: _____ **Comments:** _____

   _____

   _____

3. **Title/Author:** _____

   Publisher/Series: _____ ISBN Number: _____

   Format: _____ No. of Questions: _____

   Rating: _____ **Comments:** _____

   _____

   _____

   _____

4. **Title/Author:** _____

   Publisher/Series: _____ ISBN Number: _____

   Format: _____ No. of Questions: _____

   Rating: _____ **Comments:** _____

   _____

   _____

5. **Title/Author:** _____

   Publisher/Series: _____ ISBN Number: _____

   Format: _____ No. of Questions: _____

   Rating: _____ **Comments:** _____

   _____

   _____

--(fold here)--

Return Address

_____

_____

_____

Postage
required

Attn: Contributions
First Aid for the USMLE Step 2
Appleton & Lange
107 Elm Street
P.O. Box 120041
Stamford, CT 06912–0041

--(fold here)--

User Survey

Contributor Name: _____

School/Affiliation: _____

Address: _____

_____

Telephone: _____

What student-to-student advice would you give someone preparing for the USMLE Step 2?

What would you change about the study and test-taking strategies listed in Section I: Guide to Efficient Exam Preparation?

Were there any high-yield facts or topics in Section II that you think were inaccurate or should be deleted? Which ones and why? What would you change or add?

What review books for the USMLE Step 2 are not covered in Section III? Would you change the rating of any of the review books in Section III? If so, which one(s) and why?

How else would you improve *First Aid for the USMLE Step 2?* Any other comments or suggestions? What did you like most about the book?

Return Address

_____

_____

_____

Postage
required

Attn: Contributions
First Aid for the USMLE Step 2
Appleton & Lange
107 Elm Street
P.O. Box 120041
Stamford, CT 06912–0041

Guide to Efficient Exam Preparation

INTRODUCTION

Study Schedule for the USMLE. . .
Study 2 months for Step 1.
Study 2 weeks for Step 2.
Study 2 days for Step 3.
Abbreviated Study Schedule for the USMLE. . .
Study 2 weeks for Step 1.
Study 2 days for Step 2.
Bring #2 pencil for Step 3.
. . . according to many wise physicians
who have passed the entire USMLE series

While it may not seem so long ago that you passed the USMLE Step 1, you are now faced with the next step, the USMLE Step 2. This book is intended to help make your exam preparation easier.

USMLE STEP 2—THE BASICS

The USMLE Step 2 is the second of three examinations required for medical licensure in the United States. The USMLE is a joint program of the National Board of Medical Examiners (NBME) and the Federation of State Medical Boards (FSMB).

The purpose of the exam is "to determine if an examinee possesses the medical knowledge and understanding of clinical science considered essential for provision of patient care under supervision, including emphasis on health promotion and disease prevention" (Step 2 General Instructions, Content Description, and Sample Items). Translated, this means that the Step 2 is a much more clinically oriented exam than Step 1.

Format

This multiple-choice examination is administered over a 2-day period. It includes approximately 720 items divided into four test booklets. On each day of the examination, one booklet is administered in the morning and another in the afternoon. Three hours are allotted for the completion of each booklet.

Question Types

You will be familiar with the one-best-answer items and matching sets that were used in Step 1. However, the most recent Step 2 examinations (August 1994 and March 1995) included a new question format. A clinical scenario is given, and you are asked to choose several answers to one question, such as "What are the 5 best tests to order to diagnose this problem?" Your five answers are coded under one question, and partial credit may be given. Whether this type of question will become a standard part of the exam is unknown. It may have been an experimental question. As this represented only a handful of questions, you should continue to concentrate on the traditional one-best-answer items and matching sets.

UNITED STATES MEDICAL LICENSING EXAMINATION™

USMLE Step 2 is administered to students and graduates of U.S. and Canadian medical schools by the
NATIONAL BOARD OF MEDICAL EXAMINERS® (NBME®)
3750 Market Street, Philadelphia, Pennsylvania 19104-3190.
Telephone: (215) 590-9700

STEP 2 SCORE REPORT

US•MLE
United States
Medical
Licensing
Examination

Doe, Jane
123 Main St.
Apt #85
Anytown, USA 12345-6789

USMLE ID: 4-008-786-8

Test Date: September 1994

The USMLE is a single examination program for all applicants for medical licensure in the United States; it replaces the Federation Licensing Examination (FLEX) and the certifying examinations of the National Board of Medical Examiners (NBME Parts I, II, and III). The program consists of three steps designed to assess an examinee's understanding of and ability to apply concepts and principles that are important in health and disease and that constitute the basis of safe and effective patient care. **Step 2** is designed to assess whether an examinee possesses the medical knowledge and understanding of clinical science considered essential for the provision of patient care under supervision, including emphasis on health promotion and disease prevention. Results of the examination are reported to medical licensing authorities in the United States and its territories for use in granting an initial license to practice medicine. The two numeric scores shown below are equivalent; each state or territory may use either score in making licensing decisions. These scores represent your results for the administration of Step 2 on the test date shown above.

PASS	This result is based on the minimum passing score required by USMLE-recommended pass/fail result or may establish a different passing score for their own jurisdictions.

233	This score is determined by your overall performance on the examination. The score scale is based on the performance of students in medical schools accredited by the Liaison Committee on Medical Education (LCME) who took the NBME comprehensive Part II examination for the first time in September 1991 and were in their final year of medical school at the time they were tested. The scale was defined to have a mean of 200 and a standard deviation of 20 for this group. Most examinees receive a score between 140 and 260. A score of 167 is required by USMLE to pass Step 2. The standard error of measurement (SEM)+ for this scale is five points.

88	This score is also determined by your overall performance on the examination. A score of 82 on this scale is equivalent to a score of 200 on the scale described above. A score of 75 on this scale, which is equivalent to a score of 167 on the scale described above, is required by USMLE to pass Step 2. The SEM+ for this scale is one point.

+ Your score is influenced both by your general understanding of clinical science and by the specific set of items selected for this Step 2 examination. The SEM provides an estimate of the range within which your scores might be expected to vary by chance if you were tested repeatedly using similar tests.

INFORMATION PROVIDED FOR EXAMINEE USE ONLY

The Performance Profiles below are provided solely for the benefit of the examinee. The USMLE will not provide or verify the Performance Profiles for any other person, organization, or agency.

USMLE STEP 2 PERFORMANCE PROFILES

PHYSICIAN TASK PROFILE	Lower Performance	Borderline Performance	Higher Performance
Health & Health Maintenance			XXXXXXXXX*
Understanding Mechanisms of Disease			XXXXXXXXX
Diagnosis			XXXXXXX
Principles of Management			XXXXXXXXX

ICD-9 DISEASE PROCESS PROFILE

	Lower Performance	Borderline Performance	Higher Performance
Normal Growth & Development; Principles of Care			XXXXXXXXXXXXX
Infectious & Parasitic Diseases			XXXXXXXXXXX
Neoplasms			*
Immunologic Disorders			XXXXXXXXXXXXX
Diseases of Blood & Blood-Forming Organs			XXXXXXXXXXXXX
Mental Disorders			XXXXXXXXXXXXX
Diseases of the Nervous System & Special Senses			XXXXXXXXXXX
Cardiovascular Disorders			XXXXXXXX*
Diseases of the Respiratory System			XXXXX*
Nutritional & Digestive Disorders			XXXXXXXXXXXXX
Gynecologic Disorders			XXXXXXXXXX*
Renal, Urinary & Male Reproductive Systems			XXXXXXX*
Disorders of Pregnancy, Childbirth & Puerperium		XXXXXXXXXXXXXX	
Musculoskeletal, Skin & Connective Tissue Diseases		XXXXXXXXXXXXX	
Endocrine & Metabolic Disorders			XXXXXX*
Injury & Poisoning		XXXXXXXXXXXXX	

DISCIPLINE PROFILE

	Lower Performance	Borderline Performance	Higher Performance
Medicine			XXXXXXX*
Obstetrics & Gynecology			XXXXXXXXX*
Pediatrics			XXXXXXXXXXX
Preventive Medicine & Public Health			XXXXXXX*
Psychiatry			XXXXXXXXXXX
Surgery			XXXXXXX

The above Performance Profiles are provided to aid in self-assessment. Performance bands indicate areas of relative strength and weakness. Some performance bands are wider than others; the wider bands indicate less measurement precision than the narrower bands. An asterisk indicates that your performance band extends beyond the displayed portion of the scale.

The shaded area defines a borderline level of performance for each content category. Borderline performance is comparable to a HIGH FAIL/LOW PASS on the Total Test.

Additional information concerning the topics covered in each content area can be found in the *USMLE Step 2 General Instructions, Content Outline, and Sample Items.*

149VC223

Scoring and Failure Rates

The Step 2 score report should be received 6 to 8 weeks after taking the exam. It includes your pass/fail status, two numeric scores, and a performance profile.

Both scores are determined by your overall performance on the examination. The first score scale is based on the performance of the September 1991 NBME Part II examinee group. The scale was defined to have a mean of 200 and a standard deviation of 20 for this group. *A score of 167 is set by USMLE to pass Step 2.*

The second score scale defines a score of 82 as equivalent to a score of 200 on the scale described above. *This second score scale requires a score of 75 to pass Step 2.*

Since the first administration of the USMLE Step 2 in September 1992, the pass rate for NBME-registered first-time test takers has been 91–94%. This is higher than the Step 1 pass rate (see Table 1 on page 6).

Defining Your Goals

In approaching Step 2, it is useful to define your personal goals. This will allow you to make appropriate preparation and study plans.

Factors to consider:

■ Does your school require passing scores on Step 1 and 2 to graduate?

Naturally, everyone wants to pass Step 2. However, the ramifications of failing differ. According to the American Association of Medical Colleges (AAMC) Curriculum Directory (1992–93), 89 LCME-accredited medical schools require students to take the Step 2 examination, while 45% require a passing score for graduation. In any case, you must eventually pass all three steps of the USMLE to become a licensed physician in the United States.

■ Does your school use USMLE scores for class rank or other honors, such as admission into AOA?

Most schools do not use USMLE scores for class rank. However, scores may be used as criteria for other honors, such as scholarships, awards, and admission into honor societies, such as AOA.

■ Will your residency program use this score in the selection process?

As some resident applicants will not have Step 2 scores available at the time of interviewing, Step 2 scores are difficult to use in comparing applicants. However, some more competitive programs, particularly those that use the early match system, may require these scores. It is best to talk to interns in your field of choice to see if this is your situation.

TABLE 1. 1993–1994 Step 2 Administrations

Number Tested and Percent Passing

	September 1992		March 1993		September 1993	
	# Tested	% Passing	# Tested	% Passing	# Tested	% Passing
NBME-Registered Examinees						
First-Time Takers	8,508	94%	5,310	93%	9,269	94%
Repeaters	356	69%	617	72%	354	60%
NBME Total	8,864	93%	5,927	91%	9,623	92%
ECFMG-Registered Examinees						
U.S. Citizens	524	28%	647	21%	689	28%
Foreign Citizens	4,849	40%	6,622	42%	7,927	44%
ECFMG Total	5,373	39%	7,269	40%	8,616	43%

	September 1993		March 1994		August 1994	
	# Tested	% Passing	# Tested	% Passing	# Tested	% Passing
NBME-Registered Examinees						
First-Time Takers	9,269	94%	6,555	91%	9,833	92%
Repeaters	354	60%	751	67%	564	56%
NBME Total	9,623	92%	7,306	89%	10,397	90%
ECFMG-Registered Examinees						
First-Time Takers	6,141	49%	9,494	42%	7,380	47%
Repeaters	2,475	29%	4,043	23%	4,691	32%
ECFMG Total	8,616	43%	13,537	37%	12,071	41%

NBME = National Board of Medical Examiners.
ECFMG = Educational Commission for Foreign Medical Graduates.

How a particular residency program will use your scores varies. The Universal NRMP Application Form only asks when you took Step 1 or Step 2. However, many programs use their own application forms. Some ask that you fill in your scores, while others even go so far as to ask for a copy of your scores. Others will simply ask if you passed, and a few don't ask at all.

■ Will your scores be used in the future, ie, for fellowships?

Many students feel that Step 2 is less important because it often cannot be used by residency selection committees. However, you should also consider your long-term goals. Your Step 2 score will be more important than your Step 1 score if you are applying for a competitive fellowship.

■ Will this reflect your strengths or weaknesses compared to Step 1?

For most, but not all, medical students, Step 1 closely reflected academic performance in the basic science years. Likewise, Step 2 should reflect your clinical performance during your third year of medical school. For those who believe their clinical skills to be more representative of their abilities, Step 2 can be a way to show this strength. However, Step 2 may also show one's weaknesses.

When to Take the Exam

The exam is offered in early fall and early spring. In recent years, the pass/fail rates have been similar for the fall and spring exams.

Some schools may require their students to take the earlier exam. So, the percentage of students at each school taking a particular exam will vary. However, if given the choice, the student must weigh several factors.

Timeline for Studying

While this is a very personal decision, most students spend much less time studying for this exam compared to the time spent for Step 1. Most are limited by clinical responsibilities as fourth-year students. This is particularly true for the fall test-takers who may also be doing important clinical rotations to get recommendations for residency applications.

Try talking to fourth-year students or interns who recently took the exam. The amount of time spent studying varies. Some students may take a month of vacation to study. Others may not study at all. The majority try to study as much as their clinical responsibilities allow, a few days to several weeks before the exam.

Studying *can* improve your score. And, of course, studying can also help your clinical performance as a medical student and ultimately, as a physician.

In the Fall	In the Spring
Advantages: • Scores are available to residencies. This may be required in some competitive residencies. This may also allow you to show your clinical strength, particularly if you scored below your expectations on Step 1. • Your memory of the subject material from 3rd year clinical rotations will be fresher. This may be particularly important for rotations that are often not repeated in the 4th year, such as Ob-Gyn and Peds. • You can "get it over with." This will allow you to concentrate on residency aplications and to enjoy your second semester. • You will have an opportunity to take the test in the spring, in case you are ill or fail. In general, however, there will be little benefit in taking the test over to improve your score, unless extenuating circumstances caused you to score lower than expected.	Advantages: • Scores are not available to residencies. This may be to your advantage if you know standardized exams are one of your weaknesses. In most cases, not having Step 2 scores should not hurt you. But then again, it can't help you either. • You will have more clinical experience to use in taking the exam. • You can avoid the pressure of studying for this exam while trying to finish residency applications. This will allow you to concentrate on important clinical rotations during the first semester.
Disadvantages • If you score poorly, your scores will be available to residencies.	Disadvantages • Some schools will not allow you to graduate if you fail. Others will allow you to start your internship. In either case, you must take the exam the following fall if you fail. • You have to study in the second semester of your last year of medical school. Many students have "senioritis" by this time.

Study Methods

By now, you should have a good sense of which study techniques work best for you. The goal should be to use your limited study time effectively.

Your *first* step should be to assess your weaknesses. You may have a good idea based on grades from your clinical rotations. It is also very helpful to take a comprehensive practice exam that breaks down questions by subjects. Tests are also available for each subject, allowing you to score each subject individually. This will allow you to concentrate on your weak areas. This is particularly important because of your limited time and resources.

Study Materials

For several reasons, most students buy and use far fewer study materials for Step 2. Fourth-year medical students, in general, have less time to study for this exam. Some are simply more confident in their ability to pass with a good score. There are also fewer books for Step 2 on the market. Furthermore, students are less likely to invest in review and test books which will not be used again, particularly in subjects unrelated to their residency of choice. For example, unless you are planning to become a surgeon, purchasing a surgery review text this late in your medical school career may be a poor investment.

An informal survey of one medical school showed that the majority of students *used* between one and five different books. Students often used review texts or practice questions that were designed to help study for rotation exams. Be willing to *share* study materials. Most students only *purchased* one to three books. These were usually a comprehensive review book, a comprehensive book of practice questions, or review/practice questions in weak subjects.

Remember that the quality of available material is highly variable:

- Review books may be too detailed for review or cover material not emphasized on the exam. Step 2 is much more clinically oriented, making it more difficult to summarize in a review book.
- Practice question books may contain outdated questions and answers. Even "revised" editions with recent publication dates contain questions written years ago. Be careful with answers pertaining to more recent topics, such as AIDS and the role of *H pylori* in gastric ulcers.
- Practice question books may contain poorly written questions, having a different format or focus than that of the USMLE. Infrequently, answers may be incorrect.
- Explanations for practice questions vary in quality. Some merely repeat information gathered from the question. Some may explain why a particular answer is right, but do not explain why another answer is wrong. The best explanations give you an *understanding* of the topic.

Section 3 of this book provides ratings on Step 2 study materials, as well as major texts and handbooks to be used on clinical rotations or for boards review.

Test-Taking Strategies

By now, you should be familiar with your skills in taking standardized exams. However, Step 2 is different than Step 1 in many respects.

You have approximately 1 minute per question. This is more time than was available on Step 1. However, *Step 2 questions tend to be much longer.* Most Step 2 questions begin with a description of a patient or a clinical situation. Sometimes, this involves several paragraphs with related laboratory data. It can therefore be very helpful to read the last sentence to see what you will be asked. In some cases, the given information has no bearing on the question, except to introduce the topic. For example, you may have a long paragraph describing the history, physical findings, and evaluation of a hypertensive patient. The question may then simply ask which diseases hypertension is a risk factor for.

In general, matching sets are found at the end of each booklet. Many test-taking "experts" suggest doing these first. Most often, you will either know the answer to these questions or you won't. There may be less reasoning involved. Thus, you can quickly finish these questions. Remember that each question has the same amount of worth. Thus, whether you spend 5 minutes on a question or 10 seconds, only a correct answer counts!

How Step 2 Differs From Step 1
The strong clinical orientation of Step 2 makes this exam quite different from Step 1. There is less emphasis on minutia and a greater emphasis on diagnosis and management. While you will still need a large factual database, your clinical reasoning will also be very important. You will often be given several answers that are all part of the clinical diagnosis or management, but you must choose the first step to take or the most important therapeutic intervention.

Step 2 questions tend to be much longer than those of Step 1. You are often given clinical vignettes, with patient history, physical findings, and laboratory tests to sort out. Not all the information given will be pertinent to choosing the correct answer, so part of your job will be to figure out what is relevant and what is not. The most important difference between Step 1 and 2? Most medical students find Step 2 much easier. This means that most medical students spend less time studying for Step 2 and less time worrying about Step 2 when it's over. Most medical students come out of the exam feeling more secure than they did after going through the agony of Step 1.

How to Approach Each Subject
The Step 2 General Instructions, Content Description, and Sample Items section includes a broad content outline. Most students will not find this particularly helpful. However, it is a more manageable list than found for Step 1. It is worth skimming.

This exam integrates material organized in three "dimensions." The first dimension, "disease process," covers not only disease, but also what is "normal."

The second dimension, "physician task," includes promoting health and health maintenance, understanding mechanisms of disease, establishing a diagnosis, and applying principles of management. The third dimension, "population group," emphasizes conditions and disease processes specific to particular age groups or populations.

This means that the exam is not organized by subjects. However, in more practical terms, it is easier to study from six traditional subjects: medicine, surgery, pediatrics, obstetrics-gynecology, psychiatry, and public/preventive health.

Overall, the examination emphasizes *common* diseases and their *initial* diagnosis and management.

Medicine

This is such a broad subject that many students find it difficult to tackle. Zero in on your weak areas. There is a definite emphasis on cardiovascular and pulmonary diseases, including related risk factors such as smoking and HTN. However, you will also see a fair number of questions in subspecialties, such as GI, endocrine, infectious disease, and rheumatology.

Surgery

Some students believe that there are fewer questions on surgery. This is partly because many surgical questions border on internal medicine. In addition to understanding medical diagnosis and treatment, you should know surgical indications. You do not need to know surgical techniques.

Pediatrics

The key here is to not be fooled by what is normal! There is an emphasis on normal growth and development. You should be familiar with basic developmental milestones, immunization schedules, respiratory infections, and newborn disorders.

Obstetrics-Gynecology

Many medical students in the past have felt that a heavy emphasis was placed on Ob-Gyn. Partly this is because Ob-Gyn questions are easier to identify with the "G_P_" introductions. This also may be due to the fact that this is a weak area for many medical students who have limited experience in Ob-Gyn, perhaps only one clinical rotation. If this is the case for you, Ob-Gyn is worth studying. Many clinical vignettes begin with, "G_P_ woman presents with. . . ." Just because a woman is pregnant, however, does **not** mean that every illness is related to her pregnancy. Remember that a pregnant woman can have an appendicitis! In gynecology, emphasize your study on vaginal bleeding, STDs, and gynecologic cancers.

Psychiatry

The emphasis is on diagnosis of major depression, bipolar disorder, schizophrenia, and personality disorders. This does include child and adolescent disorders, such as ADHD and conduct disorder, as well as sexual disorders. On the last exam, there were no questions on developmental theories of Freud, Erikson, or Piaget! Another major emphasis is on pharmacotherapy. In addition to drugs used in the treatment of psychiatric disorders, you should know about overdose and withdrawal symptoms of alcohol and other street drugs.

Public/Preventive Health

There *is* an emphasis on health promotion and disease prevention, as stated in the purpose of the exam. This includes a mix of epidemiology/biostatistics, preventive health measures, occupational diseases, poisonings, ethics, and knowledge of risk factors. Many students do not study this discipline because it is felt to be "easy" or "common sense." Remember, though, that each question gained in public health is equal to a question in any other section in determining overall score.

Other Topics

You should be proficient at laboratory interpretation, basic EKG reading, and chest x-ray reading. There is little to no emphasis on medication dosages, biochemical pathways, and management of diseases for which there is controversy or a lack of a standard of care.

High-Yield Facts

Presenting history	Chest pain with radiation to jaw, neck, arm, or back; diaphoresis, weakness, nausea, dyspnea, apprehension.
Possible physical findings	Depends on site of infarction; tachycardia with hypertension or bradycardia with hypotension; JVD; new systolic murmurs.
Laboratory findings	Cardiac enzymes: order plasma CK and CK-MB on admission and serially; (1) CK-MB appears 4 to 6 hr after infarction, peaks within 1 day, declines within 3 days. (2) LDH_1 peaks within 2 to 3 days, remains elevated 1 to 2 weeks.
ECG findings	Varies, but classically, peaked T waves, ST-segment elevation, new Q waves, T-wave inversion.
Treatment	1. Pain control: sublingual NTG, morphine, or meperidine. 2. Oxygen: by nasal cannula or face mask, may need to intubate. 3. Reperfusion: thrombolysis within 6 hours with streptokinase or TPA; consider angioplasty. 4. Adjuvant therapy: heparin, aspirin, beta-blockers.

Patient presentation	Dyspnea, orthopnea, paroxysmal nocturnal dyspnea, diaphoresis, cyanosis, fatigue.
Possible physical findings	Sinus tachycardia; pink, frothy sputum; rales; S_3 gallop.
CXR	Pulmonary venous congestion, cardiomegaly, Kerley A & B lines, peribronchial cuffing.
Diagnosis	By measuring capillary wedge pressure (> 20 mm Hg).
Treatment	1. Oxygen. 2. Morphine. 3. Loop diuretics (ie, furosemide). 4. Nitrates. 5. Digoxin. 6. Treat underlying condition.

Internal Medicine

HIGH-YIELD FACTS

Presenting history	Hx of coagulation abnormality, recent surgery, immobilization, or oral contraceptive use.
Symptoms	Dyspnea, sudden chest pain, apprehension, cough.
Findings	ABG shows PaO$_2$ below 90 mm Hg, ECG may show sinus tachycardia, CXR will often be normal.
V/Q scan	Negative scan will rule out PE; equivocal results require further diagnostic work-up, ie, impedance plethysmography, Doppler ultrasound, or pulmonary angiography.
Treatment	Oxygen to correct hypoxemia, thrombolytic therapy with streptokinase, urokinase, or TPA for resolution of present thrombi, IV heparin for prophylaxis against further emboli, pulmonary embolectomy rarely done.

INTERNAL MEDICINE—CAUSES OF PNEUMONIA

Infants	Viral.
Young adults	*M pneumoniae.*
Adults	*S pneumoniae.*
Community-acquired	*S pneumoniae.* *M pneumoniae.* *H influenzae.* Empiric TX with erythromycin.

INTERNAL MEDICINE—PNEUMONIA

Type of Infection	Clinical Findings	Laboratory and Imaging Findings, Other Comments
Bacterial	Varies, but classically with high fever, chills, and productive cough.	Segmental or lobar infiltrate for pneumococcal pneumonia.
Atypical	Not generally fulminant, constitutional sxs, plus a nonproductive cough, HA, myalgias, arthralgias.	Complement fixation titer for *Mycoplasma,* immunofluorescence for *Legionella,* specific antibodies for TWAR.

Viral	Generalized body aches, malaise, and dry, nonproductive cough.	Hazy infiltrates; acute and convalescent sera.
Fungal	Asymptomatic or chronic dry, nonproductive cough.	Blastomycosis in the Midwest. Histoplasmosis in central and eastern United States. Coccidioidomycosis in Southwest.

INTERNAL MEDICINE—ANEMIA

Low MCV	Most common causes: Iron deficiency, thalassemia, anemia of chronic disease, sideroblastic anemia, and lead intoxication.
Normal MCV	Hemolysis, aplastic anemia, acute hemorrhage, renal failure.
High MCV	B_{12} or folate deficiency.

INTERNAL MEDICINE—LAB ANALYSIS OF ANEMIA

	RI	G:E	Bilirubin (mg/dL)	Examples
Blood loss	1%	3:1	<1	External bleeding.
Hypoproliferative	<2%	3:<1.5	<1	Fe def., inflammation, low E-PO
Hemolytic	>3%	3:>3	>1	Hereditary spherocytosis.
Ineffective erythropoiesis	<2%	3:>3	>1	Folic/B_{12}, thalassemias.

INTERNAL MEDICINE—MICROCYTIC ANEMIAS

Abnormality	Ferritin	Serum iron	TIBC
Iron deficiency	↓ (first finding).	↓	↑
Chronic disease	N/↑	↓	↓

Sideroblastic anemia	N/↑	↑	N
Thalassemia	N/↑	N/↑	N

INTERNAL MEDICINE—MICROCYTIC ANEMIAS (LOW MCV)

Iron deficiency anemia	Initial: **dec. serum ferritin;** next: dec. serum iron and inc. TIBC; late: hypochromic, microcytic cells.	Most common cause of anemia, usually due to blood loss, also consider postgastrectomy malabsorption or pregnancy.
Thalassemia	Dec. MCV with normal serum iron, ferritin, and TIBC.	More common among Mediterranean and Asian individuals.

INTERNAL MEDICINE—MACROCYTIC ANEMIA

Folate deficiency	Elderly on "tea and toast" diets, alcoholism, malabsorption, oral contraceptives or anticonvulsant drugs, increased utilization (hemolytic anemia or pregnancy).
B$_{12}$ deficiency	Pernicious anemia, gastrectomy, pancreatic insufficiency, GI bacterial overgrowth, ileitis or ileal resection, intestinal parasites.

INTERNAL MEDICINE—DIABETES

	IDDM	NIDDM
Synonyms	Type 1, juvenile onset.	Type 2, adult-onset.
Pathogenesis	Pancreatic beta-cell destruction (absolute lack of insulin).	Abnormal insulin secretion and peripheral insulin resistance.
Clinical features	Child or adolescent, normal to wasted body habitus, polydipsia, polyuria, weight loss despite increased appetite.	Middle-aged, obese, polydipsia, polyuria, weight gain.

Acute complications	Ketoacidosis.	Hyperosmolar, nonketotic coma.
Treatment	Diet, insulin.	Weight loss, diet, sulfonylureas, insulin.

INTERNAL MEDICINE—HYPONATREMIA

Volume status	Common causes	Treatment
Hypovolemia	GI losses, renal losses, third-space losses.	Isotonic saline.
Hypervolemia	Liver disease, heart failure, nephrotic syndrome, renal insufficiency.	Water restriction.
Isovolemia	Glucocorticoid insufficiency, advanced hypothyroidism, nausea, pain, or emotional stress, potassium depletion and diuretics, psychogenic polydipsia, drugs, SIADH.	Water restriction.

Note: Too rapid correction of sodium level may cause central pontine myelinolysis and permanent neurologic damage.

INTERNAL MEDICINE—POTASSIUM DISTURBANCES

Potassium disturbance	Rapid correction	Slow correction
Hyperkalemia	CaCl or $D_{10}W$ + regular insulin.	Sodium polystyrene sulfonate or dialysis.
Hypokalemia	KCl IV, monitor heart with replacement > 20 mEq/hr, check STAT potassium every 2 hr.	KCl orally.

Note: Correction of hyperkalemia is to protect heart from the effects of potassium (bradycardia, prolongation of AV conduction, AV block, vertricular fibrillation).

INTERNAL MEDICINE—IV FLUIDS

Isotonic normal (0.9%) saline	ECF replacement, correction of hyponatremia and whenever a tendency for metabolic alkalosis is present.
Half normal (0.45%) saline	Sodium maintenance, gastric fluid replacement.

LR	Best ECF replacement, good for replacing GI losses, sufficiently "physiological" to not affect the body's acid-base balance significantly.	
D₅W	Replacement of insensible water loss, correction of hyperosmolar dehydration.	

INTERNAL MEDICINE—RHEUMATOLOGY

Osteoarthritis	Insidious onset; morning stiffness; little to no effusion, tenderness, or redness; bony, hard, and cool joints; affects DIP joints (Heberden's nodes) and PIP joints (Bouchard's nodes).	No signs of inflammation (normal ESR and CRP). X-ray shows spurring and bony proliferation.
Rheumatoid arthritis	Prodromal symptoms of malaise, fever, weight loss; symmetric joint swelling, redness, and tenderness; wrists and MCP's involved; swan-neck deformity and boutonniere deformity; extra-articular manifestations include subcutaneous nodules, pleural effusion, pericarditis, and vasculitis.	Increased ESR, CRP; rheumatoid factor positive in 90%, increased serum gamma globulins. X-ray shows joint erosions, narrowed joint spaces, and juxta-articular osteoporosis.
SLE	Women in childbearing age with systemic sxs of fever, malaise, and weight loss; malar rash, mucosal ulcers, alopecia, arthritis, and renal disease.	+antinuclear antibody. +anti-double strand DNA. +anti-Smith nuclear Ag. Rule-out drug-induced lupus (procainamide, hydralazine, isoniazid).
Scleroderma	Diffuse scleroderma or CREST (calcinosis, Raynaud's phenomenon, esophageal dysmotility, sclerodactyly, and telangiectasias).	Mild anemia. +antinuclear antibody.

INTERNAL MEDICINE—PULMONARY TUBERCULOSIS

High-risk groups	HIV-positive individuals, IV drug abusers, immuno-suppressed patients, foreign-born persons from high prevalence countries (ie, Africa, Far East, Central or South America), medically underserved low-income populations, residents of long-term care facilities (ie, nursing homes).	

HIGH-YIELD FACTS

Internal Medicine

Internal Medicine *(left margin)*

HIGH-YIELD FACTS *(left margin)*

Screening	Members of high-risk groups should be screened, as well as close contacts with persons known or suspected to have TB. Screening with 5 tuberculin units of purified protein derivative (PPD), injected intracutaneously, is the preferred test. Patients with signs or sxs of pulmonary TB should have CXR done.
Signs and symptoms	Fatigue, fever, night sweats, anorexia, dry, nonproductive cough, dyspnea, pleuritic chest pain, and hemoptysis.
Diagnosis	Positive acid-fast smear.
Treatment	For uncomplicated pulmonary TB infections, begin with 2 months of multi-drug therapy, including isoniazid, rifampin, and pyrazinamide, plus ethambutol if isoniazid resistance is suspected. Pending culture results, INH and rifampin may be continued for the final 4 months. Many different regimens may be used, but therapy is based on the principle that multi-drug therapy should be used to overcome drug resistance to a single agent.
Complications of therapy	Hepatotoxicity.

INTERNAL MEDICINE—HYPERSENSITIVITY REACTIONS

	Type	Mediators	Examples
I	Anaphylactic.	IgE.	Anaphylaxis.
II	Cytotoxic.	IgG, IgM.	Hemolytic anemia, Goodpasture's.
III	Immune complex.	Ag-Ab.	Serum sickness, SLE.
IV	Cell-mediated (delayed).	T cells.	TB, contact dermatitis, transplant rejection.

Internal Medicine Notes

begin on page 22

_____

_____

_____

_____

_____

_____

_____

_____

_____

_____

Internal Medicine

HIGH YIELD FACTS/IMPORTANT TOPICS FROM INTERNAL MEDICINE ROTATION

1.

2.

3.

4.

5.

6.

7.

8.

9.

10.

HIGH-YIELD FACTS

HIGH-YIELD FACTS

Internal Medicine

OBSTETRICS AND GYNECOLOGY—ABORTIONS

	Definitions	Clinical Correlation
Definition	Spontaneous loss of the products of conception before 20 weeks of gestation.	Most due to fetal genetic abnormalities; should treat for Rh disease.
Threatened	Spontaneous vaginal bleeding before 20 weeks' gestation.	Reassurance.
Inevitable	Bleeding plus crampy lower abdominal pain plus cervical dilation.	Admit, symptomatic relief for pain, ultrasound to ensure abortion complete plus F/U pregnancy tests.
Incomplete	Passage of tissue in the presence of symptoms of inevitable abortion.	Same as "Inevitable"; monitor for complications such as hemorrhage and sepsis.
Complete	All tissue passed; cramps and bleeding abate with contraction of cervical os; all symptoms of pregnancy disappear (negative pregnancy test).	Investigate if two or more known first trimester abortions or one second trimester abortion.
Missed	Retention of non-viable fetus in uterus for significant period of time.	Can be terminated as soon as possible.

OBSTETRICS AND GYNECOLOGY—FETAL HEART MONITORING

	Definitions	Clinical Correlation
Normal heart rate	120–160 bpm.	
Normal beat-to-beat variability	3–7 bpm.	
Absence of beat-to-beat variability		Associated with fetal acidosis (pH < 7.20); also associated with analgesics and sedatives or fetal sleep state.
Tachycardia	FHR > 160 bpm.	Associated with intrauterine, infection, hypoxia, or thyrotoxicosis.
Bradycardia	FHR < 114 bpm.	Not as significant.

Sinusoidal pattern	Oscillations of > 25 bpm.	Nonspecific indication of fetal compromise.
Early decelerations	Begins with onset of contraction with same duration, nadir coincides with the peak of contraction, heart rate returns to baseline after contraction.	Innocuous condition which usually reflects uterine contractions causing changes in fetal heart rate; thought to be vagus response due to compression of fetal head in birth canal but must check for prolapsed umbilical cord.
Late decelerations	Onset usually after onset of contraction.	Associated with uteroplacental deficiency; first response is to place mother on side (to relieve pressure of uterine weight on aorta, vena cava, and iliacs); then give oxygen by face mask, stop oxytocin, give tocolytic, and monitor maternal blood pressure to exclude maternal hypotension; if pattern persists, get fetal scalp pH; values lower than 7.2 will prompt surgery.
Variable decelerations	Independent of uterine contraction, rapid drop and return to baseline.	Often indicative of fetal umbilical cord compression; perform vaginal exam for prolapsed umbilical cord; try changing maternal position (to side); if pattern persists, monitor fetal pH (associated with respiratory acidosis) or immediate delivery (cesarean) indicated.

OBSTETRICS AND GYNECOLOGY—DIFFERENTIAL DX OF BLEEDING DURING PREGNANCY

Spontaneous abortion of fetus	Most commonly associated with genetic defects of the fetus; will often present before 20 weeks of gestation with cramping, mild uterine bleeding; if cervix is changing, abortion is inevitable; tx by delivery of fetus; if complete fetus is not recovered, must evacuate by D&C.

Obstetrics and Gynecology

HIGH-YIELD FACTS

Contact bleeding	Rich vascular supply of the cervix causes it to be more vulnerable to trauma (as during intercourse); bleeding is usually mild and painless without cramping; diagnosis of exclusion.
Cervical effacement and dilatation	Bleeding can occur as cervix starts to change; usually bleeding is mild, at or near term, and is preceded by expulsion of cervical mucous.
Placenta previa	Painless vaginal bleeding in late second or early third trimester; hemorrhage may be brisk; U/S will show location of placenta; *avoid digital exam;* get L/S ratio for fetal lung maturity; fetus delivery by cesarean.
Placental abruption	Vaginal bleeding, uterine tenderness, and cramping; U/S may show abruption; lab may show abnormal CBC and coagulation parameters; if abruption is mild, pregnancy monitored expectantly; if severe, then fetus must be delivered; maintaining maternal hemodynamics is priority; DIC is most lethal complication.
Ectopic pregnancy	Severe pain early in pregnancy, h/o sexual activity, especially unprotected sex; check pregnancy test, U/S often shows fetus; tx is evacuation of fetus.

OBSTETRICS AND GYNECOLOGY—MENOPAUSE

Definition	Normal cessation of menstruation in a woman with previously normal menstrual cycles; often occurs after a perimenopausal period during which menstrual cycle changes in length.
Age of onset	Average age: 51 years, normal range of 45 to 55 years.
Physiology	Due to failure of normal follicular development.
Symptoms	Hot flushes, night sweats, insomnia, and changes in vaginal tract secondary to hypoestrogenism.
Therapy	Estrogen replacement to prevent the morbidity associated with decreased estrogen levels: osteoporosis and increased risks of cardiovascular disease; HRT may be associated with an increase of breast cancer but therapy is recommended unless there is a direct contraindication (ie, previous breast Ca, liver dz).

Gonorrhea	*Neisseria gonorrhea*	Mucopurulent D/C from urethra or vagina, pharyngitis, abnormal uterine bleeding, 2 to 10 days after intercourse.	Gram stain and culture show gram negative diplococci.	Ceftriaxone or ciprofloxacin; treat also for *Chlamydia*.
Chlamydia	*Chlamydia trachomatis*	Mucopurulent cervical D/C 7 to 14 days postintercourse, dysuria, often asymptomatic.	Tissue culture, PCR immunoassays, fluorescent immuno-antibody assay.	Doxycycline.
Syphilis	*Treponema pallidum*	Primary: chancre 10 to 90 days after direct contact. Secondary: skin rash, lympha-denopathy, condylomata lata. Tertiary: asymptomatic.	Clinical exam and positive serology.	Benzathine penicillin.
Herpes	Herpes simplex	Burning pain, pain or tingling with flu sx followed by eruption of grouped vesicles 3 to 7 days after contact.	Cytologic stain with multinucleated cells, tissue culture.	Acyclovir for outbreaks.
Condyloma acuminata (warts)	Human papilloma-viruses	Warty growths.	Visual, may biopsy for confirmation.	Ablation, increased risk of cervical and vulvar cancer.
HIV	Human immuno-deficiency virus	Fatigue, lymphadenopathy, wt. loss, diarrhea, night sweats, cough.	ELISA confirmed by Western blot.	Symptomatic AZT.
Trichomonas vaginalis	Protozoa	Yellow-green vaginal D/C, strawberry cervix.	Wet mount showing flagellated organisms.	Metronidazole.

OBSTETRICS AND GYNECOLOGY—BREAST CANCER

Epidemiology	Most common cancer affecting women in the United States, incidence is one in eight.
Symptoms	Few early, later skin dimpling, eczema, bloody D/C from nipples, fixation of breast, distortion of nipple, reddening and ulceration of skin and bone pain (metastases).
Histology	Most common is adenocarcinoma from ductal or lobular epithelium.

Management   Evaluate patient with complete cancer work-up.

Survival   Dependent on stage plus presence of hormone receptors (positive receptors for estrogen and for progesterone indicate better prognosis).

Treatment   Surgery, ± radiation, ± tamoxifen (if estrogen receptors are positive), ± chemotherapy; 50% of patients with breast cancer die from their disease.

OBSTETRICS AND GYNECOLOGY—ADRENAL DISEASES

Cushing's syndrome   Central fat placement, cushingoid features, menstrual irregularities, and hirsutism; diagnosis with dexamethasone suppression test; treat with surgery (if tumor); GnRH blocks secretion of gonadotropins from pituitary.

Congenital adrenal hyperplasia   Deficiencies of 21-hydroxylase or 11-B-hydroxylase inherited as autosomal recessives; infants born with ambiguous genitalia.

OBSTETRICS AND GYNECOLOGY—GESTATIONAL DIABETES

Risk factors   Hx prior stillbirth, prior fetus greater than 9 lb, morbid obesity, glucosuria, multiple diabetic family members.

Complications   Increased risk of fetal malformation and stillbirth; can cause macrosomia of the fetus with consequent complications of delivery secondary to dystocia or cephalopelvic disproportion.

Screening   1 hr post-prandial glucose at 24 to 48 weeks.

Treatment   Glucose control with exogenous insulin.

OBSTETRICS AND GYNECOLOGY—GYNECOLOGICAL CANCERS

Disease	Age, Risk Factors	Presenting Symptoms	Evaluation
VIN	HPV.	Vulvar pruritis, chronic irritation, whitish raised mass lesions.	Acetic acid wash and biopsy.

Vulvar carcinoma	65 to 70 yr old, postmenopausal.	Vulvar pruritis, red or white, ulcerative or exophytic lesions.	Biopsy, if confirmed, CSR, IVP, cystoscopy, proctoscopy as needed; squamous cell most common.
CIN	Younger than 30, carcinogen exposure, cigarette smoking, HPV.	Annual Pap smear.	Pap smear, colposcope, or cervical conization.
Cervical carcinoma	Very young to very old, CIN, HPV, multiple sex partners, cigarette smoking, immunocompromised.	No classic presentation; postcoital bleeding or abnormal uterine bleeding.	Biopsy; squamous cell most common; clear cell associated with DES.
Leiomyoma	Any age.	Pelvic pain, bleeding, and pressure symptoms; consider leiomyosarcoma in woman with rapidly enlarging uterine mass and postmenopausal bleeding, unusual vaginal discharge, and pelvic pain.	Abdominopelvic exam and pelvic ultrasound.
Endometrial hyperplasia	Unopposed estrogen (see endometrial cancer).	Abnormal bleeding, especially over age 35.	Endometrial sampling; most common cystic, adenomatous, and atypical adenomatous.
Endometrial cancer	Most postmenopausal; risk factors include exogenous estrogen alone, hx chronic anovulation, obesity, postmenopausal, late menopause (>55 yr).	Abnormal bleeding, especially postmenopausal bleeding.	Endometrial sampling; prognosis based on histological grade.
Ovarian cancer	Postmenopausal women in 5th and 6th decade; risk factors include low parity, dec. fertility, delayed childbearing; long-term suppression of ovulation (ie, by OCPs) has protective effect against ovarian cancer.	Symptoms appear late.	Usually fatal.

Presenting symptoms	Pregnancy with uterine size/date discrepancy, exaggerated sxs of pregnancy, painless bleeding early in 2nd trimester, tissue fragments passed through cervical os; other sxs include visual disturbances, nausea, vomiting, preeclampsia, proteinuria.
Evaluation	U/S shows "snowstorm" appearance.
Management	Order β-HCG, CXR, Hb/HCT, and blood type/Rh; treat complete GTD with curettage; incomplete GTD with same or induction of labor; older women may undergo hysterectomy; F/U with β-HCG.

COMPARISON OF COMPLETE AND PARTIAL GESTATIONAL TROPHOBLASTIC DISEASE

Complete GTD	Partial GTD
Syncytiotrophoblasts	Cytotrophoblasts.
Hydropic placental villi	Degeneration of the placenta.
NO fetus	Abnormal fetus.
Paternal 46,XX	69,XXY.
Most common, most malignant potential	Malignant potential.

Obstetrics and Gynecology Notes

begin on page 32

Obstetrics and Gynecology

HIGH-YIELD FACTS

HIGH YIELD FACTS/IMPORTANT TOPICS FROM OBSTETRICS AND GYNECOLOGY ROTATION

1.

2.

3.

4.

5.

6.

7.

8.

9.

10.

PEDIATRICS—DEVELOPMENT

Age	Language	Motor	Other
6 mo	Babbles.	Sits well unsupported.	Recognizes strangers.
9 mo	Uses "Dada/Mama."	Crawls, uses pincer grasp.	Starts to explore environment.
1 yr	1 to 3 words.	Walks.	Stranger and separation anxiety.
2 yr	Pronouns, 2- to 3-word phrases.	Walks up and down steps, holds cup.	Parallel play.
3 yr	Routine use of sentences.	Pedals tricycle.	Group play.

PEDIATRICS—ORDER OF PUBERTAL DEVELOPMENT

Male	Testicular enlargement.
	Pubic hair development (axillary hair follows).
	Penile growth.
	Peak of height spurt.

Female	Breast development.
	Pubic hair development (axillary hair follows).
	Peak of height spurt.
	Menarche.

PEDIATRICS—NEONATAL JAUNDICE

Physiologic jaundice	Bilirubin peaks at 3rd day of life (5th day in premature infants).	Consider phototherapy or exchange transfusion.
Breast milk jaundice	Bilirubin peaks during second week of life.	Stop breast feeding for 1 to 2 days.
Pathologic	Jaundice (bilirubin > 5 mg/dL) on 1st day of life, bilirubin level increases greater than 0.5 mg/dL/hr, peak bilirubin is greater than 13 mg/dL in term infants.	Consider: hemolysis, internal hemorrhage, infection, Crigler-Najjar, blood group incompatibility, RBC dysfunction, thalassemias.

Complete transposition of the great arteries	Aorta arises from the RV and pulmonary trunk arises from LV.	Cyanosis, S_2 appears loud and single; CXR: classic "egg-shaped" heart.
Tetralogy of Fallot	VSD, overriding aorta, pulmonary stenosis, RVH.	Harsh systolic ejection murmur at left sternal border due to PS, single S_2, CXR: classic "boot-shaped" heart.

VSD	Disappearance of S_1, mid-diastolic rumble at apex, soft systolic ejection murmur at ULSB.	RVH, LVH.
ASD	Mid-diastolic rumble at LLSB.	RAD, RVH, later pulmonary HTN.
PDA	Mid-diastolic at apex, systolic ejection at apex.	LAH, LVH.

Brudzinski sign	Bending head forward produces flexion of the lower extremities.			
Kernig sign	Not being able to extend the knee when hip is flexed.			
	Pressure	**Leukocytes (/uL)**	**Protein (mg/dL)**	**Glucose (mg/dL)**
Normal	50–180 mm H_2O.	< 4 (70% lymphs, 1–3% PMNs).	20–45.	> 50 or 75% blood glucose.
Acute bacterial meningitis	Increased.	100–60,000 PMNs predominate.	100–500.	Decreased.
Tuberculous meningitis	Usually increased.	10–500 early: PMNs predominate late: lymphs predominate.	100–500.	Decreased.

HIGH-YIELD FACTS

Pediatrics

Viral meningitis	nL, or slightly increased.	PMNs early, mononuclear cells later.	20–100.	nL, or decreased in some viral diseases.

PEDIATRICS—BACTERIAL MENINGITIS

Pathogen	Epidemiology	Clinical Findings	Lab Findings	Treatment	Prophylaxis
H influenzae, type B	Under 5 years of age, especially < 2 years.	Frequently followed URI, associated with arthritis, cellulitis.	Gram stain CSF shows gram-negative rods; often positive blood Cx.	Cefotaxime, ceftriaxone, cefuroxime or ampicillin and chloramphenicol.	Rifampin, *H influenzae* vaccine.
N meningitidis	Infants and young children; patients with complement deficiency.	Morbilliform, petechial, or purpuric rash, shock.	Gram stain CSF shows gram-negative diplococci.	Same as *H influenzae.*	
S pneumoniae	Children with deficiencies of humoral immunity or asplenic patients; post-traumatic.	Frequently follows URI, otitis, sinusitis, pneumonia.	Gram stain CSF shows gram-positive diplococci.	Penicillin or ampicillin; if resistant, vanco, chloramphenicol, cefotaxime.	Abx prophylaxis for sickle cell patients and asplenic; pneumococcal vaccine.
Group β strep	Neonates.		Gram stain CSF shows gram-positive cocci in chains.	Amp/gent or amp/cefotaxime.	Abx prophylaxis of pregnant women or neonate.
M tuberculosis	High-risk geographic group or ethnic group.	Onset is gradual; TB pneumonia often present, sxs are encephalopathic type.	Positive tuberculin skin test; acid-fast bacilli in CSF.	INH and rifampin, plus a 3rd and 4th drug (PZA, streptomycin, ethambutol).	INH to PPD+ and contacts with TB.
Aseptic meningitis	Nonbacterial inflammation of the meninges, most commonly enterovirus		No bacteria, mycobacteria, protozoans, or yeasts in CSF.	Usually benign and self-limited; acyclovir for herpes.	

	Definition	Clinical Findings	Cause	Treatment	Complications
Acute OM	Onset of new infection.	Ear pain, pulling at ear, ± fever, irritability, associated with URI, erythema of TM, bulging, absent landmarks	*S pneumonia, H influenzae, M catarrhalis;* infants: above, plus *S aureus* and *C trachomatis.*	Initial tx: amoxicillin x 10 days. If no response in 40 hr, Augmentin, cefaclor, Pediazole, or TMP/Sulfa; recheck after 10-day course of therapy for evidence of middle ear effusion.	Hearing loss of 20–3 dB, which can persist for several mo; rupture of TM; mastoiditis.
Recurrent acute OM	3 episodes of AOM within 6 mo or 4 episodes within 1 yr.	Same as AOM.	Underlying problem: chronic sinusitis, allergy, immune defect, anatomic defect, adenoidal hypertrophy; passive smoke exposure; bedtime bottle propping.	Amoxicillin or sulfisoxazole × 6 mo; if this fails, referral to ENT for tympanostomy tube placement.	Same as AOM.
Persistent OM with effusion (serous otitis, secretory otitis, "glue ear")	Middle ear effusion that fails to resolve with therapy within 6 weeks.	Decreased hearing (conductive hearing deficit), ear fullness, ear popping, opaque, dull TM with decreased mobility, air bubbles behind the TM.	Mechanical obstruction (cleft palate, adenoidal hypertrophy), allergy, attendance at day care, passive smoke exposure, same pathogens as AOM, plus *S epidermidis* and diphtheroids.	Abx against β-lactamase producers or TMP–SMX for 4 to 6 weeks; myringotomy and tympanostomy tube placement if effusion persists > 3 mo despite therapy or hearing loss; adenoidectomy if above fails.	Cholesteatoma, erosion of ossicles, hearing loss.

| Chronic OM | Middle ear effusion persisting longer than 12 weeks despite therapy, or irreversible damage to middle ear structures. | Chronic foul-smelling otorrhea, hearing loss, granulation tissue on TM which is thickened, immobile TM, tympanosclerosis. | *Pseudomonas* and *S aureus* are common pathogens. | Refer to ENT for surgical tx; may need parenteral antibiotics based on culture results. | Same as persistent OM. |

PEDIATRICS—CAUSES OF SMALL BOWEL OBSTRUCTION

Small bowel obstruction Manifested by bilious vomiting; common causes include adhesions, appendicitis, intussusception, inguinal hernia, Meckel's diverticulum, and malrotation (volvulus).

PEDIATRICS—COMMON GASTROINTESTINAL DISEASES

	Epidemiology	Findings	Complications	Treatment
Gastro-esophageal reflux	Common first year of life.	24-hr esophageal pH monitoring is definitive diagnostic test.	Cause of neonatal apnea.	Elevating head after feedings, bethanechol and metoclopramide to increase lower esophageal tone, H2 blockers and antacids; surgical: Nissen fundoplication.
Hypertrophic pyloric stenosis	More common in male and full-term infants.	Onset of projectile nonbilious vomiting begins 2 to 4 weeks of life; gastric olive-shaped mass, "string sign" on barium UGI, U/S for identification of hypertrophied muscle.	Weight loss, hypokalemic metabolic alkalosis, dehydration.	Restoration of fluid and electrolyte balance, pyloromyotomy.

Duodenal atresia (complete obstruction) and stenosis (partial obstruction)	More common in premature and infants with Down syndrome.	Abdominal x-ray shows "double bubble."	Complete obstruction: polyhydramnios; bilious vomiting, abdominal distention; in neonates, there might be failure to pass meconium.	Restoration of fluid and electrolyte balance, nasogastric suction to relieve obstructive sxs, surgery: definitive tx.
Intussusception	More common in children between 6 to 18 mo old; seen in patients with cystic fibrosis and HSP.	Acute onset of colicky intermittent abd. pain; child drawing up the knee to ease the pain; passage of "currant jelly" stool (blood and mucus clot); sausage-shaped mass is palpable in the upper abdomen.		Enema: not only confirms DX but with appropriate hydrostatic pressure may reduce the intussusception. Surgery: when reduction with enema is unsuccessful.

PEDIATRICS—NEWBORN HYPOGLYCEMIA

Serum glucose	Premature infant ≤ 25 mg/dL. Term infant ≤ 35 mg/dL first 72 hr, or < 40 to 45 mg/dL 72 hr after birth.
Causes	1. Persistent hyperinsulinemia in infant of a diabetic mother. 2. Erythroblastosis fetalis. 3. Beckwith-Wiedemann syndrome. 4. β-sympathomimetic drugs used for tocolysis.
Symptoms	Epinephrine release: tachycardia, diaphoresis, flushing, tachypnea. Cerebral hypoglycemia: stupor, seizures, coma, lethargy, jitteriness, poor feeding.
Treatment	1. Infant alert and without contraindications for oral feeding should be encouraged to drink carbohydrate solutions. 2. Infant not capable of oral feedings should receive IV glucose (10% dextrose solution).
Prognosis	With seizure activity, prognosis is poor, associated with abnormal neurointellectual development.

Preterm infants

In most cases, should be immunized at the usual chronologic age; vaccine dosages should not be decreased; if exposed to hepatitis B in utero, should receive HBIG within 12 hr of birth and the HBV; if chronic respiratory dz, should be immunized against influenza at 6 mo of age.

Pregnancy

Only vaccines routinely recommended for administration during pregnancy are tetanus and diphtheria; influenza and pneumococcal vaccine can be given if high risk for serious illness; HBV can be given if indicated; all live-viral vaccines (MMR, OPV) are contraindicated, except when exposure is highly probable and the dz poses a greater threat than the vaccine; women immunized with MMR should wait 3 mo after vaccination to become pregnant.

Immunodeficient and immunosuppressed children

Live virus and live bacterial vaccines are contraindicated; siblings and other household contacts should not receive OPV but can receive MMR.

Children receiving immunosuppressive therapy—influenza vaccine can be given 3 to 4 weeks after therapy is discontinued and live virus vaccine 3 mo after therapy is discontinued.

Children with HIV infection—MMR is recommended regardless of clinical status due to severe measles infections with fatalities in these children.

Asplenic children

Important pathogens in these children are *S pneumoniae, H influenzae* type B, and *N meningitidis;* therefore, polyvalent pneumococcal vaccine, HiB, and quadrivalent meningococcal vaccines are recommended; daily antimicrobial prophylaxis is recommended; PenVee is usually recommended.

Children with seizure or family history of seizures

These children are at an increased risk for having convulsions after pertussis (DTP) or measles (MMR) vaccine; a family history of seizures is NOT a contraindication to pertussis or measles vaccination.

Anaphylactic allergy to eggs	MMR, MR, influenza.
Anaphylactic allergy to neomycin	MMR, MR, OPV.
Anaphylactic allergy to streptomycin	OPV, IPV.

PEDIATRICS—RESPIRATORY INFECTIONS

Infection	Clinical Findings	Susceptible Ages	Season	Agent	DX	TX
Common cold (URI)	Clear rhinorrhea, nasal congestion, sneezing, mild fever, cough.	All ages.	Throughout the year, peak in the fall and spring.	Rhinovirus is most common.		Treatment for viral URI is symptomatic.
Sinusitis	Fever, headache, purulent rhinorrhea, nasal congestion lasting more than 10 days, chronic cough, pain to palpation over frontal and maxillary sinuses.	All ages.	Throughout the year.	*S pneumoniae, H influenzae, M catarrhalis*	Sinus x-ray.	Amoxicillin × 10 days, or × 21 days if chronic.

HIGH-YIELD FACTS

Pediatrics

41

Strepto-coccal pharyngitis	Fever, sore throat, head-ache, abd. pain, exudative tonsillitis, tender anterior cervical nodes.	None.	None.	Group A beta hemolytic strep, *S pyogenes*.	Throat culture, rapid strep screen.	Penicillin for 10 days; treat-ment is im-portant to prevent com-plications (glomeru-lonephritis, acute rheumatic fever).
Infectious mononu-cleosis	Malaise, fatigue, headache, fever, sore throat, splenomegaly, ant. and post. cervical nodal tenderness.	None.	None.	EBV.	Positive monospot test, antibodies to EBV, atypical lymphocytes.	
Acute epiglottitis	Rapid onset of fever and sore throat, respira-tory distress, stridor, drooling, sitting forward with mouth open, cherry red epiglottis.	2 to 7 yr.	None.	*H influenzae* type B.	Neck x-ray shows "thumb" sign; if high degree of suspicion of epiglottitis, the x-ray should not be done, and the diagnosis should be confirmed by direct laryn-goscopy in a controlled setting.	Nasotracheal intubation, admit to ICU, IV antibiotics to cover β lactamase producing *H influenzae*.
Croup	Hoarseness, barking cough, fever, stridor, URI.	6 mo to 3 yr.	Fall.	Parainfluenza-virus	Neck x-ray: "steeple sign."	Cool mist, aerosolized racemic epinephrine.

Pediatrics

HIGH-YIELD FACTS

Bron-chiolitis	Cough, wheezing, dyspnea, crackles, flaring of nasal alae.	2 to 6 mo, rare after 2 yr of age.	Late fall and winter.	RSV most common; adenovirus; parainfluenza virus 1 and 3.	Immunofluorescent techniques to identify the virus in nasal secretions.	Supportive measures: IV hydration, oxygen, aerosolized ribavirin if due to RSV.
Bacterial pneumonia	Fever, shaking chills, cough, chest pain, crackles, decreased breath sounds.	*S pneumoniae* all ages; *H influenzae* children under age 5.	Late winter to early spring.	*S pneumoniae, H influenzae* type B.	CXR: consolidation; increased WBC, positive blood cx.	*S pneumoniae:* (a) PCN or (b) amp and cefotaxime in infants. *H influenzae:* (a) cefuroxime or (b) erythromycin and sulfisoxazole.
Myco-plasma pneumonia	Moderate fever, malaise, sore throat, nonproductive cough.	5 to 15 yr old.	Fall.	*Mycoplasma pneumoniae.*	CXR: perihilar lymphadenopathy and interstitial infiltrate of lower lobe involvement.	Erythromycin or tetracycline as an alternative for patients > 9 yr of age.

Pediatrics

HIGH-YIELD FACTS

_____

_____

_____

_____

_____

_____

_____

_____

_____

HIGH YIELD FACTS/IMPORTANT TOPICS FROM PEDIATRICS ROTATION

1.

2.

3.

4.

5.

6.

7.

8.

9.

10.

HIGH-YIELD FACTS

Pediatrics

PREVENTIVE MEDICINE—REVIEW OF KEY TERMS

Prevalence	Number of *current* cases per given population at a given *point* in time.
Incidence	Number of *new* cases per population during a given *period* of time.
Relative risk	Ratio of the incidence of disease in subjects with a risk factor to the incidence of disease in subjects without a risk factor. Mainly used in cohort studies

$$\frac{I_{exposed}}{I_{not\ exposed}}$$

$$\frac{\dfrac{a}{a+c}}{\dfrac{b}{b+d}}$$

$$I_{exposed} - I_{unexposed}$$

Attributable risk	Estimate of the excess disease or other outcome due to that risk factor I(exposed)—I(not exposed).
Odds ratio	Ratio of the odds of exposure to the risk factor given disease to the odds of exposure to the risk factor given no disease. Mainly used in case-control studies ad/bc.

PREVENTIVE MEDICINE—TESTING TERMINOLOGY

Sensitivity

Probability of test being positive when disease is present.

True pos. ÷ disease positive.

True pos. ÷ (true pos. + false neg.).

$$\frac{a}{a+c}$$

Specificity

Probability of test being negative when disease is absent.

True neg. ÷ disease negative.

True neg. ÷ (true neg. + false pos.).

$$\frac{d}{b+d}$$

		Disease	
		Present	**Absent**
Test Results	**Positive**	a	b
	Negative	c	d

Positive predictive value	Proportion of patients with a positive test who have the disease or probability of disease being present when test is positive.
	True pos. ÷ test pos.
	True pos. ÷ (true pos. + false pos.).
	$$\frac{a}{a+b}$$

Negative predictive value	Proportion of patients with a negative test who do not have the disease or probability of disease being absent when test is negative.
	True neg. ÷ test neg.
	True neg. ÷ (true neg. + false neg.)
	$$\frac{d}{c+d}$$

Null hypothesis	Assumption that the observed difference between two groups of patients studied is *due to chance,* rather than due to one of the groups having received treatment.

Type I error	Rejecting the null hypothesis when it is true.

Type II error	Not rejecting the null hypothesis when it is false.

p-value	Probability that the difference occurred by chance alone; probability of a type I error.

Power	Probability of detecting a real difference when one actually exists; 1-probability of a type II error.

PREVENTIVE MEDICINE—TYPES OF STUDIES

Study	Description	Calculations
Cohort	Prospective study of a group to determine the development of an outcome (no intervention is applied).	Mainly used to calculate incidence, relative risk, and attributable risk.
Cross-sectional	Measures the association of a risk factor and disease of a group of subjects at a single point in time.	Mainly used to calculate prevalence, sensitivity, specificity, and odds ratio.

PREVENTIVE MEDICINE—TYPES OF STUDIES *(continued)*

Case-control	Retrospective study of groups with (case) and without (control) disease to compare past exposure to a risk factor.	Mainly used to calculate odds ratio. Cannot calculate prevalence or incidence.

PREVENTIVE MEDICINE—CATEGORIES OF PREVENTION

Category	Definition
Primary	Prevention of disease.
Secondary	Early detection and treatment of disease.
Tertiary	Limitation of disability and rehabilitation.

PREVENTIVE MEDICINE—OCCUPATIONAL HAZARDS

Hazard	Source of Exposure	Risk
Silicon dioxide	Molding process.	Silicosis.
Asbestos	Insulation.	Asbestosis, associated with malignant mesothelioma.
UV and infrared light	Welding process.	Skin and eye ("flash") burns.
Cadmium	Electroplating process, batteries.	Pneumonitis, pulmonary edema.
Cotton dust	Textile manufacturing.	Byssinosis.

PREVENTIVE MEDICINE—CORONARY HEART DISEASE

Risk factors include smoking, hypercholesterolemia, HTN, obesity, and OCP use among women over age 35 and who smoke.

PREVENTIVE MEDICINE—STROKE

Risk factors include old age, hypertension, smoking, coronary heart disease, atrial fibrillation, diabetes mellitus, and oral contraceptive use.

A significant risk factor for lung, larynx, mouth, pancreas, and bladder cancers; chronic obstructive lung disease, coronary heart disease, stroke, and peripheral vascular disease.

PREVENTIVE MEDICINE—CANCER RISK FACTORS AND SCREENING

Cancer	Major Risk Factors	Screening
Lung	Smoking.	None for the general population.
Breast	Age > 50 years, personal or family history of breast cancer, nulliparity, or first child after age 30. From a clinical standpoint, all older women should be considered at risk.	*Breast self-exam* every month for women age 20 and older. *Clinical breast exam* every 3 years for women ages 20 to 39, every year for women ≥ age 40. *Mammography* every 1 to 2 years for women ages 40 to 49 and annually for women ≥ age 50.
Colon and rectum	Personal or family history in first-degree relatives of polyps or colorectal cancer, a family history of polyposis syndromes, and a personal history of inflammatory bowel disease.	*Digital rectal exam* annually, for men and women age 40 and older, stool blood test annually for men and women age 50 and older, sigmoidoscopy exam once every 3 to 5 years, for men and women > age 50.
Cervix	Early age at first vaginal intercourse, multiple sexual partners, cigarette smoking, HPV types 16, 18, 31, and 33.	Women who have been sexually active, or have reached age 18 or older; annually; after three or more satisfactory, consecutive, normal annual exams, may be performed less frequently.

Adapted, with permission, from American Cancer Society Textbook of Clinical Oncology, 1991, 155.

HIGH-YIELD FACTS

Preventive Medicine

PREVENTIVE MEDICINE—TETANUS

History of Absorbed Tetanus Toxoid Doses	Clean, Minor Wounds	All Others
Unknown or < 3	Td.	Td and TIG.
≤ 3	Td only if more than 10 years since last dose.	Td only if more than 5 years since last dose.

PREVENTIVE MEDICINE—SPECIFIC POISON ANTIDOTES

Substance	Antidote
Acetaminophen	Acetylcysteine.
Pit viper venom, black widow spider venom	Antivenin.
Organophosphates and carbamate insecticide poisons	Atropine.
Lead and other heavy metals	Calcium EDTA.
Iron	Deferoxamine.
Digoxin	Digoxin antibody.
Mercury	Dimercaptosuccinic acid.
Methanol and ethylene glycol	Ethanol.
Benzodiazepines	Flumazenil.
Chemically induced methemoglobinemia	Methylene blue.
Opioids (narcotics)	Naloxone.
Carbon monoxide	Oxygen.
Copper, lead, mercury, arsenic	Penicillamine.

Anticholinergic poisoning	Physostigmine.	
Organophosphate insecticide poisoning	Pralidoxime.	
Isoniazid poisoning	Pyridoxine.	

PREVENTIVE MEDICINE—SPIDERS AND SCORPIONS

	Habitat	Symptoms	Treatment
Black widow spider	Woodpiles, sheds, basements, April to October.	Sharp pain at site, cramping pain of abdomen and extremities.	Antivenin and pain relief with hot tub bath, calcium gluconate, and methocarbamol.
Brown recluse spider	Midwest, also South and Southwest.	Mild stinging to intense local pain with bullae and erythema, can cause ischemic necrosis.	If mild, no treatment necessary; if severe, parenteral glucocorticoids; dapsone and antivenin considered experimental.
Scorpion	Most are nonlethal; dangerous species in Southwest.	Immediate burning sensation, then paresthesias locally then whole extremity.	If mild, cold compresses and mild analgesics; if severe, constriction bands, antivenin, and supportive TX.

Preventive Medicine

HIGH-YIELD FACTS

_____

_____

_____

_____

_____

_____

_____

_____

_____

HIGH YIELD FACTS/IMPORTANT TOPICS FROM PREVENTIVE MEDICINE ROTATION

1.

2.

3.

4.

5.

6.

7.

8.

9.

10.

PSYCHIATRY—DSM

Axis 1	Clinical syndromes.
Axis 2	Personality disorders and developmental disorders.
Axis 3	Physical disorders.
Axis 4	Severity of psychosocial stressors.
Axis 5	Global assessment of functioning.
Mini-mental status examination	Orientation, registration, attention and calculation, recall, language.

PSYCHIATRY—BIOLOGIC THEORIES OF MENTAL ILLNESS

Depression	Decreased norepinephrine and serotonin.
Schizophrenia	Excessive dopaminergic activity.
Anxiety	Interference of benzodiazepine-GABA receptor and increased norepinephrine in locus ceruleus.

PSYCHIATRY—DIFFERENTIAL DIAGNOSIS OF SCHIZOPHRENIA

Schizophrenia	Characteristic psychotic symptoms of hallucinations or delusions for at least 6 months, including an active phase for at least 1 week.
Schizophreniform disorder	Same as schizophrenia except duration of symptoms at least 1 month but less than 6 months.
Brief (reactive) psychotic disorder	Same as schizophrenia except occurs in individuals under severe stress and symptoms last at least 1 day but less than 1 month.
Schizo-affective disorder	Schizophrenia with symptoms of a mood disorder, better premorbid functions and prognosis than schizophrenia.
Paranoid personality disorder	Similar to schizophrenia but lacks hallucinations and formal thought disorder.

Schizoid personality disorder	*Withdrawn and aloof* but lacks chronically disordered thinking of schizophrenia.
Schizotypical personality disorder	*Odd or eccentric* thinking and communication but lacks frank psychosis of schizophrenia.

PSYCHIATRY—DEPRESSION SYMPTOMS (SIG E CAPS)

S	**S**leep disturbance.
I	**I**nterest decrease or loss.
G	**G**uilt (self-esteem).
E	**E**nergy (libido) decrease or loss.
C	**C**oncentration (decision making) decrease or loss.
A	**A**ppetite disturbance.
P	**P**sychomotor agitation or retardation.
S	**S**uicidal and depressed mood and affect.

PSYCHIATRY—DIFFERENTIAL DIAGNOSIS OF MOOD DISORDERS

Dysthymia	Chronic, rather than episodic, depression of mild to moderate severity.
Cyclothymia	Periods of depression and hypomania with briefer mood swings and less severe symptoms than in bipolar disorder.
Bereavement	Normal process with many symptoms similar to depression but lacks guilt about actions at the time of death or hallucinations, may last up to 1 year.
Postpartum blues	Normal condition of tearfulness, fatigue, anxiety, and irritability, lasting only a few days after childbirth.

Postpartum psychosis
Usually experienced within days to first 8 weeks after delivery; suspicion, confusion, incoherence, irrational statements, and obsessive concerns about the baby's health; in a psychiatric emergency, hallucinations may tell patients to kill themselves or their babies.

PSYCHIATRY—DEPRESSION VS GRIEF

Depression
Irrational erosion of self-esteem, perplexed as to feelings of sadness (not obviously related to a loss).

Grief
Seldom persists beyond 2 months, seldom needs medication, no associated suicidal tendencies or neurovegetative signs.

PSYCHIATRY—BORDERLINE VS NARCISSISTIC PERSONALITY DISORDERS

Borderline
Unstable relations with overidealized devaluation, labile affect, self-mutilation, empty and bored, frantic about abandonment, impulsive with drugs, sex, and money, binge eating can resemble bipolar depression.

Narcissistic
Special sense of entitlement, grandiose, hates or esteems other people, reacts to criticism with rage or shame or humiliation.

PSYCHIATRY—DELIRIUM VS DEMENTIA

Delirium
Acute organic brain syndrome characterized by a clouded state of consciousness, usually of rapid onset, fluctuating course, and short duration; recent memory loss, visual hallucinations, disoriented especially to time, and generalized EEG slowing.

Dementia
Chronic organic brain syndrome usually of insidious onset and slow, persistent deterioration; recent and remote memory loss; often abnormal neuroimaging studies; consistent mental status decline; cortical dysfunction (apraxia or agnosia); attempts to conceal; gives near-miss answers.

Psychiatry

HIGH-YIELD FACTS

Panic disorder	Sudden and unpredictable attacks of fear and apprehension with multiple physical symptoms.
Generalized anxiety disorder	Excessive anxiety about two or more particular circumstances for at least 6 months.
Obsessive-compulsive disorder	Persistent thoughts (obsessions) and repetitive behaviors (compulsions), associated with serotonin and cingulate gyrus.
Post-traumatic stress disorder	Reliving extremely traumatic events beyond 4–6 weeks after the event, results in impaired social, marital, work functions, hypervigilance, flashbacks, startle, arousal, and nightmares.
Phobia	Persistent, irrational fear resulting in avoidant behavior of the object, activity, or situation.

Somatization disorder	Multiple somatic complaints for which no physical cause can be found.
Conversion disorder	Sudden *neurologic* symptoms that have no known pathophysiological cause, ie, anesthesia of hand in "glove" distribution.
Hypochondriasis	Chronic preoccupation with fears of serious illness when no organic problems can be found.
Body dysmorphic disorder	Preoccupation with an imagined defect in the body.
Somatoform pain disorder	Pain in the absence of any physical findings or explanations.
Factitious disorder	Voluntary control of symptoms but with an *unconscious motive,* made worse by observation by another.
Malingering	Conscious willful faking of illness with a *conscious motive.*

HIGH-YIELD FACTS

Psychiatry

PSYCHIATRY—DISSOCIATIVE DISORDERS

Dissociative (psychogenic) amnesia	Forgetting information related to a traumatic event.
Dissociative (psychogenic) fugue	Sudden, unexpected travel away from one's home and family, associated with loss of memory about one's past and usually the assumption of a new identity.
Dissociative identity (multiple personality) disorder	Presence of two or more distinct personalities within a single person.
Depersonalization	Persistent or recurrent sense of estrangement, dislocation, or detachment from one's body or mind.

PSYCHIATRY—HUMAN SEXUALITY

Transvestism	Cross-dressing in a heterosexual male *for purposes of arousal.*
Transsexualism	Persistent sense of discomfort about one's anatomic sex and strong desire to change one's genitals and secondary sex characteristics.

PSYCHIATRY—CONDUCT AND DISRUPTIVE BEHAVIOR DISORDERS

Attention-deficit/ hyperactivity disorder (ADHD)	Developmentally or age-inappropriate inattention and/or hyperactivity-impulsivity, present for at least 6 months; causes social or academic disturbances, and occurs before the age of 7 years.
Oppositional defiant disorder	Often argues with adults, loses temper, deliberately annoys others, and blames others for his/her misbehavior; present for at least 6 months, causes social or academic disturbances, typically begins by age 8 and not later than adolescence.

Conduct disorder	Repetitive and persistent pattern of behavior in which the basic rights of others or major age-appropriate societal norms or rules are violated, including aggression against people and animals, destruction of property, deceitfulness or theft, and serious violation of rules, present for at least 6 months, typically seen in childhood and adolescence.
Antisocial personality disorder	Continual antisocial or criminal acts with a lack of remorse; evidence of conduct disorder seen before age 15, but diagnosis requires that the individual is at least age 18; the "con-artist" with no remorse or conscience; impulsive, not responsible or monogamous.

PSYCHIATRY—SUBSTANCE-RELATED TERMS

Abuse	Continued use in spite of knowing adverse consequences and use of the substance in situations in which use is dangerous or impairs role performance.
Dependence	Psychological and physical reliance on a substance that leads to substance-seeking behavior, an inability to stop using the substance, an increasing tolerance to its effects, and a deterioration in physical and mental health as a result of continued use of the substance.
Tolerance	Need for markedly increased amounts of the substance to achieve intoxication or desired effects, or a markedly diminished effect with continued use of the same amount of the substance.
Withdrawal	Cessation or reduction of substance use results in a substance-specific syndrome.

PSYCHIATRY—SUBSTANCES OF ABUSE

Substance	Signs and Symptoms of Use, Treatment	Withdrawal, Treatment
Alcohol	Maladaptive behavior, slurred speech, incoordination, unsteady gait, nystagmus, impairment of attention or memory, stupor or coma. Tx: varies—observation to support of ventilation, acid-base status, electrolytes, and temperature.	Tremulousness, delusions and hallucinations, seizures, delirium tremens, irritability. Tx: benzodiazepines.

Opioids

Constricted pupils, declining pulse rate, declining respiratory rate, pulmonary edema, stupor, coma, CNS depression.

Not life-threatening, sweating, goose flesh, dilated pupils, muscle and abdominal cramps, vomiting and diarrhea, increased BP, RR, HR, tremor.

Tx: naloxone (Narcan) and supportive measures.

Tx: detoxification, benzodiazepines, methadone, psychotherapy, clonidine, naltrexone.

CNS stimulant (cocaine)

Euphoria, mania, anxiety, increased BP, arrhythmias, dilated pupils, S2, coma, psychotic Sxs.

Crash: dysphoria, anhedonia, anxiety, irritability, fatigue, hypersomnolence.

Tx: phentolamine for HTN and hyperthermia, haloperidol for psychotic Sxs.

Tx: dopaminergic agonists or tricyclic antidepressants.

CNS stimulant (amphetamines)

Acute delirium, psychosis with long-term use.

Decreased CNS activity (crashing).

Tx: decreased CNS irritability (quiet setting), control psychotic Sxs with chlorpromazine.

Tx: sleep, physical and emotional support.

CNS depressants (barbiturates and benzodiazepines)

Drowsiness, coma (severe OD), memory impairment, nystagmus, paranoias, decreased muscle tone.

Life-threatening; seizures and CV collapse.

Tx: if awake, induce vomiting or perform gastric lavage; respiratory and cardiac support; if comatose, gastric lavage, alkalinize urine to increased excretion, intubation, oxygen, and respiratory and cardiac support.

Tx: substitute abused drug with a barbiturate or long-acting benzodiazepine; then taper.

Hallucinogens

Euphoria, illusions, hallucinations, confusion, dilated pupils (LSD), "bad trip" panic reaction.

No physical dependence or withdrawal symptoms, but psychological dependence may develop.

Tx: support, reassurance and talking, decreased stimulation, diazepam for severe pain; avoid antipsychotic drugs unless psychosis is severe.

PCP (angel dust)

Changes in body image, depersonalization, paranoia, unpredictable violence, increased BP, muscle spasm, tachypnea, nystagmus, rigidity, ataxis, coma leading to death.

Depression psychosis, permanent neurologic impairment.

Tx: mid to mod: quiet room with minimal stimulation, no talking.

| Cannabinoids (marijuana, hashish) | Disconnected speech, recent memory impairment, depersonalization, increased HR, decreased body temperature, conjunctival injection, amotivational syndrome with chronic use. | Irritability, insomnia, sweating. |
| | Tx: same as withdrawal Tx. | Tx: psychotherapy, behavior modification, group therapy. |

_____

_____

_____

_____

_____

_____

_____

_____

_____

HIGH YIELD FACTS/IMPORTANT TOPICS FROM PSYCHIATRY ROTATION

1.

2.

3.

4.

5.

6.

7.

8.

9.

10.

Zenker's diverticula	Treatment includes excision of redundant mucosa and myotomy.
Achalasia	Dysphagia of liquids > solids, regurgitation, and weight loss; x-ray shows megaesophagus with a "bird's beak appearance," increased risk for Ca. Treatment includes dilation or esophagomyotomy (Heller procedure).
Diffuse esophageal spasm	Substernal pain, "chest beaters"; manometry is key to diagnosis. Treatment is extended myotomy.
Scleroderma	Treatment includes diet, omeprazole, and surgery only if medical therapy is unsuccessful.
Esophageal reflux	Substernal pain, heartburn, regurgitation, worse when lying down, dx by manometry, esophagoscopy, pH measurement; can lead to Barrett's esophagus.
Barrett's esophagus	Secondary to chronic acid injury, squamous epithelium becomes columnar, 10% increased incidence of adenocarcinoma; complications include hemorrhage, incarceration, obstruction.
Boerhaave's syndrome	Vomiting, then sudden chest pain as a result of postemetic rupture of the esophagus.
Mallory-Weiss tear	Tear in lower esophagus near gastroesophageal junction, leading to acute massive UGI hemorrhage.
Esophageal benign tumors	Leiomyomas most common, dx includes barium swallow, esophagoscopy; bx contraindicated.
Esophageal malignant tumors	Squamous cell most common, adenocarcinoma second most common, associated with Barrett's. Risk factors: tobacco, alcohol, nitrosamines, achalasia, corrosive esophagitis, hot beverages, Barrett's; surgery provides the only cure, adjunctive radiotherapy and chemotherapy.

Symptoms	After large meal, severe epigastric pain radiating to the back with vomiting and retching; dehydration, tachycardia, postural dehydration.

Lab	Serum amylase, lipase, lipids, urine amylase, serum calcium, serum magnesium.
X-ray	Sentinel loop, colon cutoff sign.
Ranson's criteria initial	Age > 55, WBC > 16,000, blood glucose > 200, serum LDH > 350, AST > 250.
Ranson's criteria during 1st 24 hours	HCT falls > 10%, BUN increases > 8 mg/dL, serum calcium < 8 mg/dL arterial pO_2 < 60 mm Hg, base deficit greater than 4 mEq/L, fluid sequestration > 600 liters.
Mortality	Depends on number of above signs; if 0–2 signs, then < 2%, but if 7–8 signs, 100%.
Etiology	40% gallstones, 40% EtOH.

SURGERY—PANCREATIC ABSCESS

Symptoms	Severe acute pancreatitis which does not improve or worsen after period of improvement; fever, epigastric pain and tenderness with palpable mass.
Lab	Increased WBC, amylase nL, albumin < 2.5 g/dL, alkaline phosphatase increased.
X-ray	CT diagnostic (gas in abscess).
Therapy	Broad spectrum antibiotic, percutaneous catheter (rarely definitive tx), surgical debridement.

SURGERY—PANCREATIC CANCER

Symptoms of cancer of the head (2/3rds of cases)	Weight loss, obstructive jaundice, deep abdominal pain, back pain, palpable mass.
Symptoms of cancer of the body, tail	Weight loss, paroxysms of abdominal pain; patient sits with spine flexed (can't sleep in bed), otherwise the same as above.
Histology	80% are adenocarcinoma; early local extension and regional metastases to nodes and liver with later spread to lungs and peritoneum.

Lab	Increased alkaline phosphatase and very elevated bilirubin.
Therapy	Whipple procedure.
Mortality	Most die within 6 mo to 1 yr.

SURGERY—CROHN'S DISEASE VS ULCERATIVE COLITIS

	Crohn's Disease	Ulcerative Colitis
Bleeding	Rare.	Common.
Perianal disease	Common.	Rare.
Fistula	Common.	Rare.
Perforation	Common.	Rare.
Distribution	Segmental (skip lesions).	Continuous.
Mucosa	Cobblestone mucosa, fissures or deep ulcers, thickened bowel wall with stricture (string sign).	Serrated, pseudopolyps, loss of haustration (lead pipe sign).
Pathology	Granulomas, transmural involvement.	Microabscesses (crypt abscesses).
Treatment (medical)	Sulfasalazine, steroids, metronidazole (for treatment of perianal disease).	Sulfasalazine, steroids.
Treatment (surgical)	Segmental resection, panproctocolectomy with ileostomy.	Subtotal colectomy with ileooctostomy, panprocto-colectomy with permanent ileostomy, proctocolectomy with distal rectal mucosectomy and ileal pouch-anal anastomosis.
Complications	Incidence of colorectal or small bowel Ca is greater than in general population but less than for U.C.; ischiorectal, and perianal fistulas.	Toxic megacolon, colonic perforation, hemorrhage, colon Ca.

Surgery

HIGH-YIELD FACTS

History	Epigastric pain shifting to RLQ, accompanied by anorexia and vomiting.
Physical exam	Slightly elevated T (in the absence of perforation or abscess), pain on palpation over McBurney's point, guarding, rebound tenderness; peristalsis is normal or reduced.
Lab	Moderate leukocytosis, UA usually nL, but a few leukocytes and erythrocytes may be present.
X-ray	Localized RLQ ileus, air-fluid levels, or increased soft tissue density (50% of patients).
Differential diagnosis	Regional ileitis, PID, gastroenteritis, ruptured ovarian cyst, diverticulitis.
Complications	Perforation, peritonitis, appendiceal abscess.
Treatment	Appendectomy (high false positive rate).

	Juvenile	Familial
Distribution	More common in the colon than the small bowel.	Multiple adenomatous polyps throughout the large bowel.
Pathology	Hamartoma (rarely progressing to adenoma).	Adenoma.
Malignant potential	Rare.	Common.

HIGH-YIELD FACTS

Surgery

SURGERY—DIVERTICULUM (DEFECT IN MUCOSA, SUBMUCOSA, AND MUSCULARIS)

Zenker's (true)	Esophageal.	Dysphagia, halitosis, reflux, gurgling in throat, metallic taste.	Surgical (myotomy or excision); complications rare.
Meckel's (true)	Fetal remnant of yolk sac.	Occurs in 1 to 3% of population with low incidence of sx, can be dangerous in peds population where gastric mucosa remnants can cause exsanguination, cellulitis at umbilicus pathognomonic.	Surgical.
Colon (usually false)	Most often involves sigmoid colon, only affects mucosa and submucosa.	50% incidence, herniation then defects (blood supply) through circular muscularis layer either with hypermotility or aging/illness, associated with decreased fiber diets.	

SURGERY—DIVERTICULOSIS (SECONDARY TO COLONIC DIVERTICULUM)

Symptoms	Local abdominal pain (mild to severe, steady or crampy), change in the rate of bowel movements in elderly, presentation can be insidious, palpable mass occasionally on PE, tenderness, signs of peritonitis.
Diverticulitis	Infection of diverticulum with peridiverticular inflammation, abscess formation, can lead to peritonitis/obstruction, differential dx: Ca, appendicitis, Crohn's disease, mesenteric insufficiency.
Imaging	CT.
Therapy	Medical: increase fiber in diet, antibiotics for microperforations. Surgical: excision and reanastomosis.
Complications	Bleeding and diverticulitis.

Primary	Peritonitis in absence of GI perforation, occurs in cirrhotics, nephrotics, SLE, after childhood splenectomy.
Secondary	Results from bacterial contamination from within viscera or from external sources.
Symptoms	"Acute abdomen" (abdominal pain, tenderness, guarding, rigidity, distention, free peritoneal air, decreased bowel sounds) and systemic signs (fever, chills, rigors, tachycardia, sweating, tachypnea, dehydration, oliguria, disorientation, shock). Recurrent unexplained shock usually means peritoneal sepsis, elderly and immunosuppressed can have diminished symptoms.
Lab	Increased WBC, ABG, PT/PTT, LFTs, RFTs, pan-culture.
Treatment	1. IV fluids. 2. Art line and ionotropes if indicated. 3. Abx (avoid aminoglycosides). 4. Surgery to debride and treat primary disease (ie, appendix, gallbladder) **and/or** to peritoneal lavage and drain for localized residual infection.
Prognosis	Overall mortality is 40%.

	Small Intestine	Large Intestine
Etiology	Adhesions or strangulation.	Carcinoma; most often affects sigmoid.
Diagnosis	Proximal: vomiting, abdominal discomfort, abnormal x-ray. Mid/distal: colicky pain, vomiting, constipation, obstipation, peristaltic rushes, x-ray.	Constipation, obstipation, abdominal distention, abdominal tenderness, abdominal pain, nausea, late-onset vomiting, x-rays, barium x-ray or colonoscopy for localization.

HIGH-YIELD FACTS

Surgery

| **Treatment** | Partial obstruction: expectant therapy as long as passing flatus or stool, NG tube for decompression and surgery if partial obstruction persists for several days. Complete obstruction: promptly (cannot r/o strangulation) unless many previous surgeries for obstruction, post-op, inflammatory bowel disease, abdominal carcinomatosis or radiation tx. | Surgery almost always required. |

SURGERY—STAGING OF STOMACH CARCINOMA: 50% OF LESIONS WILL BE RESECTABLE

I	Extends into but not through submucosa.
II	Into but not through muscularis propria, no nodes.
III	Same as II but with positive nodes.
IV	Through muscularis propria with positive nodes.

SURGERY—STAGING OF COLON OR RECTAL CARCINOMA: OPERABLE IN 70%, SURVIVAL RATE 35%, WIDE EXCISION WITH REGIONAL LYMPHATICS

Carcinoma in situ

A	Into but not through muscularis propria.
B	Perforates visceral peritoneum or directly invades, negative nodes.
C	Tumor of any size with metastases.

SURGERY—PNEUMOTHORAX

Spontaneous	Tall, thin 20 to 40-year-old male with history of smoking	Sx begin at rest, chest pain on affected side, increasing dyspnea, tachycardia; if pneumothorax is large, will also have decreased breath sounds, decreased tactile fremitus, and hyperresonance.
Traumatic	History of trauma, esp. iatrogenic.	Same as spontaneous.
Secondary	Previous lung disease.	Same as spontaneous.

| Tension | History of penetrating trauma, lung infection, CPR, PEEP. | Severe tachycardia, hypotension, mediastinal/ tracheal shift. |

Small, new pneumothorax	Bed rest, analgesia, follow with CXR every 12 to 24 hr for 2 days.
Small, stable pneumothorax	Follow outpatient with CXR every 24 hr.
Large pneumothorax or tension pneumothorax	Tube thoracostomy (large-bore needle in an emergency).
Recurrent, bilateral, or failure of tube thoracostomy	Thoracoscopy or open thoracotomy.

Hypovolemic	Loss of blood (hemorrhage). Loss of plasma (burn). Loss of fluid and electrolytes (external or third spacing).	PAOP declines. CO declines. SVR declines.
Cardiogenic	Dysrhythmia, pump failure, regurgitant valve failure, or rupture of intraventricular septum.	PAOP increases (unless RV infarct). CO declines. SVR increases.
Obstructive	Tension pneumothorax, pericardial disease, disease of pulmonary vasculature, cardiac tumor, mural thrombus, obstructive valvular disease.	PAOP increases in pericardial tamponade or aortic dissection, declines in pulmonary embolism. CO declines. SVR increases.
Distributive	Septic, anaphylactic, neurogenic, vasodilator, acute adrenal insufficiency.	PAOP declines or no change. CO increases. SVR declines.

HIGH-YIELD FACTS

Surgery

Symptoms	Hypotension, orthostatic changes, peripheral hypoperfusion (mottled skin on extremities), altered mental status.
Treatment	Trendelenburg position, oxygen, analgesia, catheter for urine flow, ECG monitoring, monitor CVP or PCWP, fluid replacement (0.9% NaCl), dopamine or dobutamine if hypotension persists.

Surgery Notes

begin on page 74

Surgery

_____

_____

_____

_____

_____

_____

_____

_____

HIGH-YIELD FACTS

HIGH YIELD, FACTS/IMPORTANT TOPICS FROM SURGERY ROTATION

1.

2.

3.

4.

5.

6.

7.

8.

9.

10.

High-Yield Facts

This list of high-yield topics was generated by surveying a cross-section of medical students who took the USMLE Step 2 within the past 2 years.

INTERNAL MEDICINE

1. Anemia
2. B_{12}/folate deficiency
3. Blood transfusions and complications
4. Hypercalcemia and hypocalcemia
5. Cardiac tamponade
6. Congestive heart failure
7. Connective tissue disorders, including scleroderma, rheumatoid arthritis, and SLE
8. Diabetes mellitus
9. Dyspnea—work-up and initial management
10. Electrolyte disturbances and treatment—especially hypernatremia and hyponatremia
11. Endocarditis
12. Heart murmurs—correlation to pathophysiology
13. HIV
14. Hypertension
15. Myocardial infarction
16. Pancreatic disease and cancer
17. Pericarditis
18. Physical exam signs—especially those related to cardiorespiratory disease
19. Tuberculosis

OBSTETRICS & GYNECOLOGY

1. Anovulation
2. Breast disease and cancer
3. Complications in pregnancy, including bleeding and hypertension
4. Estrogen therapy and benefits
5. Fetal monitor tracings
6. Gestational diabetes
7. Labor and delivery
8. Sexually transmitted diseases, especially *Chlamydia* and *Gonorrhea*
9. Vaginal bleeding—by far the most often cited topic, including differential diagnosis and treatment

PEDIATRICS

1. Common URIs, including the common cold, croup, and epiglottitis
2. Congenital defects, especially cardiac
3. Leukemia and lymphoma
4. Neonatal complications, including Group B *Streptococcus* infection and jaundice
5. Normal growth and development

PREVENTIVE MEDICINE

1. Alcoholism
2. Cigarette smoking
3. Drugs—signs and symptoms of use and withdrawal
4. Occupational hazards
5. Poisonings
6. Risk factors for diseases

PSYCHIATRY

1. Adjustment disorder vs post-traumatic stress disorder
2. Depression
3. Personality disorders

SURGERY

1. Appendicitis
2. Initial evaluation of acute abdomen
3. Initial management of trauma
4. Pneumothorax
5. Post-surgical care and complications
6. Pulmonary embolism

Supplement

_____

_____

_____

_____

_____

_____

_____

_____

_____

HIGH YIELD FACTS/IMPORTANT TOPICS FROM SUPPLEMENT ROTATION

HIGH-YIELD FACTS

1.

2.

3.

4.

5.

6.

7.

8.

9.

10.

Book Reviews

How to Use the Book Review Section

This section is a database of current clinical books used both for clinical rotations and for boards review.

The books are sorted into sections corresponding to the major disciplines covered in the USMLE Step 2: comprehensive, internal medicine, obstetrics & gynecology, pediatrics, preventive medicine, psychiatry, and surgery.

The books are also sorted according to their major purpose: reference textbooks, handbooks, and boards review books. The reference textbooks and handbooks are evaluated specifically for their applicability to use on the wards. We made special note of those that are also useful for boards review. On the other hand, the boards review books are evaluated specifically for their usefulness in studying for the USMLE Step 2. The ratings for these boards review books are not meant to reflect their usefulness on the wards.

Each book receives a **Rating** according to the scale below. Each entry includes the **Title** of the book, **Edition, Approximate List Price, Format** of the book, **Number of Test Questions,** the **First Author** or **Editor,** the **Series Name,** if applicable, the **Publisher,** the **Publication Year, Number of Pages,** and **ISBN Code.** The narrative section of each entry includes pros, cons, and a summary of the review.

A+	Excellent for use on the wards *or* boards review. A "must have."
A A–	Also very helpful. Worth buying.
B+ B B–	Adequate for use on the wards *or* boards review. Use these books if you already own them!
C+ C C–	Poor choice for use on the wards *or* boards review. Better books are available.
D	Not appropriate for use by medical students.

The **Rating** for reference textbooks and handbooks is based on several factors, including: cost, readability, accuracy, quality of illustrations, length, size, and appropriateness for a medical student.

The **Rating** for boards review books is based on several factors, including: cost, readability, appropriateness and accuracy, quality and number of sample questions, quality of written answers to sample questions, length, quality and number of other books available in the same discipline, and the importance of the discipline on the USMLE Step 2 examination.

Disclaimer

No material in this book, including the ratings, reflects the opinion or influence of the publisher. All errors and omissions will gladly be corrected if brought to the attention of the authors through the publisher.

Comprehensive Book Reviews

begin on page 87

Review for USMLE Step 2 $32.00 Test/800 q
National Medical Review
National Medical Series
Williams & Wilkins 1994, 329 pages, ISBN 0-683-06207-7
Pros: Contains 4 practice exams, 200 questions each. Among the test
question books, this book provides questions most similar to the actual
Step 2. Answers are well-written, explaining both the right and wrong
answers.
Cons: Though each answer lists the major topic involved, it is difficult to
assess your subjects of weakness because the questions are integrated.
Summary: Most representative of the actual Step 2 exam, this test question
book provides ample practice for the real thing.

 Appleton & Lange's Review for the USMLE Step 2 $34.95 Test/1200 q
Catlin
Appleton & Lange Review Series
Appleton & Lange 1993, 290 pages, ISBN 0-8385-0226-1
New edition available February, 1996; ISBN: 08385-26665
Pros: Includes 150 questions for each subject, plus two 300-question
comprehensive practice tests. Only test book available with questions
sectioned by topic, providing an excellent way to assess your weaknesses.
Quality of answers vary, but most are good.
Cons: Some test questions are a little harder than what will appear on
Step 2.
Summary: This is the "black book" that everybody has. Among the test
question books, provides the best means for assessing your weaknesses.
If your primary method of studying will be through test questions and one
book is all you want to buy, this is a good source to consider.

 PreTest Step 2 Simulated Examination $30.00 Test/420 q
Thornborough
PreTest Series
McGraw-Hill 1993, 178 pages, ISBN 0-07-064521-3
Pros: Consists of three sections, each containing 140 questions. Indexed for
cross-referencing by subject. Topics covered by questions similar to that
seen on Step 2.
Cons: Questions tend to be shorter and easier than the USMLE Step 2.
Summary: Good source of more practice questions. Do not be lulled into a
sense of security, though, if you find these easy to answer.

B

Rypin's Clinical Sciences Review, 16th edition

$32.95   Review/Test/408 q

Frohlich

Rypin's Series

Lippincott 1993, 431 pages, ISBN 0-397-51246-5

Pros: Review of each of the six major subjects on Step 2.

Cons: Not detailed enough in some subjects, especially pediatrics. Also gives too much low-yield information in other subjects, like Ob-Gyn. Includes essay questions, clinical cases without answers, and multiple choice questions with multiple answers—none of which conforms to Step 2 format.

Summary: All-in-one review book that may be all you need to trigger your memory of weak subjects. The questions, however, do not reflect boards format.

B⁻

The Instant Exam Review for the USMLE, Step 2

$27.95   Review/0 q

Goldberg

Appleton & Lange Review Series

Appleton & Lange 1993, 363 pages, ISBN 0-8385-4038-4

New edition available February 1996

Pros: A popular choice among busy medical students as a companion to question-and-answer books because of its rapid review of subjects. Contains very brief descriptions of symptoms, diagnosis, pathology, and treatment. Medicine subspecialties are better covered than other subjects.

Cons: Coverage too incomplete for learning about new topics, but may spark just enough memory on more familiar topics. Poor coverage of pediatrics and preventive medicine. Minimal explanations of management.

Summary: A very popular choice because of rapid readability. However, a lack of details makes this a poor choice for those who need a more complete review.

C

Clinical Sciences

$41.95   Review/243 q

Bollet

Year Book's Medical Licensure Reviews Series

Mosby-Year Book 1988, 394 pages, ISBN 0-8151-1022-7

Pros: Review of major topics all in one book. More extensive in internal medicine and Ob-Gyn. Useful charts in public health section on toxins and other occupational hazards.

Cons: Few questions and in old K-type format. Shorter sections on surgery, pediatrics, psychiatry, and public health.

Summary: Another all-in-one book. Less popular than Rypin's.

Preparation for USMLE Clinical Sciences Step 2 Booklet 1, 3rd edition

$14.00   Test/315 q

Luder
Preparation for USMLE Clinical Sciences Step 2 Series
Maval Medical Education 1995, 76 pages, ISBN 1-884083-57-9
Pros: This is the first of a series of six booklets designed for Step 2 review. The pictures are the best seen in any of the available test review books on the market. Includes scoring scale to approximate pass/fail scores.
Cons: Gross errors in typing and English grammar on every page. Short explanations attempt not to repeat information obvious from the correct answer but are thus often incomplete and do not provide much learning material.
Summary: Good source for more test questions with excellent photographs. However, poor quality of questions and explanations overall.

USMLE Success!

$18.00   Guide/0 q

Zaslau, Staff of FMSG
FMSG and Stanley Zaslau 1994, 59 pages, ISBN 1-886468-02-8
Pros: Provides advice on all three steps of the USMLE. Includes a limited number of mnemonics to use as study tools.
Cons: Mostly directed toward foreign medical graduates. Paternalistic writing style with condescending attitude.
Summary: Generally not helpful for U.S. medical students who have already passed Step 1. Might be useful to foreign medical graduates.

Internal Medicine Handbooks

begin on page 91

Clinician's Pocket Reference (Scut Monkey Handbook), 7th edition　　$24.95　　Handbook/0 q

Gomella

Appleton & Lange 1993, 680 pages, ISBN 0-8385-1222-4

Pros: Contains essential details to have on the medicine wards. Useful for nearly every other rotation as well. Helps orient medical students to the wards. Contains brief differential diagnoses, explanations of abnormal lab values, and quick reference to commonly used medications. Fits perfectly into a white coat pocket.

Cons: Provides differential diagnoses but no guidelines for making the differential or for treatment.

Summary: Easy reference to carry at all times on the wards. A must to buy.

 Manual of Medical Therapeutics (The Washington Manual), 28th edition　　$32.95　　Handbook/0 q

Department of Medicine, Washington University (Woodley)

Little, Brown Spiral Manual Series

Little, Brown 1995, 603 pages, ISBN 0-316-92433-4

Pros: Provides specifics for treatment and management. Also provides brief descriptions of pathophysiology, evaluation, and diagnosis. Includes most common diseases seen on the wards.

Cons: Just slightly too big to fit in most white coat pockets, but can be stuffed in if you're willing to compress the spiral binder.

Summary: Classic handbook for the medicine wards. Should read sections of this book relevant to your patients during spare moments on the wards. A must to buy.

 Practical Guide to the Care of the Medical Patient, 3rd edition　　$27.95　　Handbook/0 q

Ferri

Mosby-Year Book 1995, 893 pages, ISBN 0-8151-3390-1

Pros: *Practical* is the best word to describe this book. Easy-to-read approach to the management of common diseases seen on the wards. Provides interpretation of lab results and descriptions of commonly used drugs, including contraindications. May be used for quick review of medicine for the boards!

Cons: Not complete for all diseases.

Summary: Quick and easy to read. Less popular than *The Washington Manual,* but should be strongly considered. Consider using this book for studying for the boards.

Internal Medicine: Diagnosis & Therapy, 3rd edition

$26.00 Handbook/0 q

Stein
Lange Clinical Manual Series
Appleton & Lange 1993, 654 pages, ISBN 0-8385-1112-0
Pros: Similar to *The Washington Manual* with good coverage of pertinent details on diagnosis and treatment of common medical conditions.
Cons: Barely fits into a white coat pocket.
Summary: Less popular than *The Washington Manual,* but a good alternative to consider carrying on the wards.

Medical Diagnosis and Therapy, 1st edition

$26.50 Handbook/0 q

Khan et al
Lea & Febiger 1994, 772 pages, ISBN 0-8121-1602-X
Pros: Good handbook for brief discussion of diseases. Covers diagnosis, pathophysiology, and therapy.
Cons: Less practical than *The Washington Manual.* Therapy is sometimes discussed in too extensive detail.
Summary: Good alternative to consider carrying on the wards.

The Internal Medicine Companion, 1st edition

$24.95 Handbook/0 q

Ferri
Mosby-Year Book 1994, 349 pages, ISBN 0-8016-7825-0
Pros: Excellent charts and algorithms of the etiology of common diseases, differential diagnosis, classification of disease processes, diagnostic approach, therapeutic modalities, medication comparison tables, and laboratory evaluation. An easy-to-read quick reference.
Cons: Neglects details in order to provide quickest reference.
Summary: Good for quick reference, especially for differential diagnosis. However, will not provide enough detail on topics new to the reader.

Internal Medicine On Call

$22.00 Handbook/0 q

Haist et al
On Call Series
Appleton & Lange 1991, 534 pages, ISBN 0-8385-4052-X
Pros: Quick reference for the initial evaluation of the most common problems seen on call. Helps guide your thinking process. Also describes common ward procedures.
Cons: A significant portion of the book includes drugs, for which better sources are available.
Summary: Good book to guide your thought process. However, if you have limited pocket-carrying space, this is not the most important source to carry.

Harrison's Principles of Internal Medicine Companion Handbook, 13th edition

$29.50   Handbook/0 q

Isselbacher et al

McGraw-Hill 1995, 940 pages, ISBN 0-07-070910-6

Pros: Condensed version of its parent textbook.

Cons: Thick and heavy, yet does not adequately address most important topics for medical students.

Summary: Better to invest in a soft-cover reference text for the same price.

Most Common Manual for Medical Students, 2nd edition

$14.95   Handbook/0 q

Grosso

Grosso 1991, 487 pages, 0-9633354-0-5

Pros: Lists the "most common" causes, complications, and conditions seen in medicine. Small, pocket-size book.

Cons: Probably not useful, especially for the boards. If it's that common, you should see it on the wards.

Summary: Good bathroom reading material, but otherwise not helpful for the boards or the wards.

Internal Medicine Review Books

begin on page 95

B Medicine, 10th edition

$19.95   Test/700 q

Baker

Medical Examination Review Series

Appleton & Lange 1991, 255 pages, ISBN 0-8385-5771-6

Pros: Short questions with short answers. Questions often ask for the "most common" or for the "best" treatment.

Cons: Answers too brief, not giving enough information to be educational. Few questions give clinical scenarios as commonly seen on Step 2.

Summary: A good value if you want to study by simply doing more questions, but should not be considered a first-line choice for boards review.

B NMS Medicine, 2nd edition

$28.00   Review/test/500 q

Myers

National Medical Series

Williams & Wilkins 1994, 585 pages, ISBN 0-683-06233-6

Pros: Provides the essentials of each subject. Easy to read in outline form. Comprehensive review of medicine, including a comprehensive exam. Brief explanations to questions.

Cons: Not to be used as a reference book for clerkship. Includes six case studies to be used as problem-solving exercises, but are not applicable to boards.

Summary: Practice questions are excellent learning tools. Too long for quick Step 2 study but more useful for a boards-style rotation exam.

B PreTest Medicine, 7th edition

$16.95   Test/500 q

Taragin

PreTest Series

McGraw-Hill 1995, 260 pages, ISBN 0-07-052024-0

Pros: Easy to read with fairly good explanations to questions.

Cons: Includes K-type questions. Covers various sub-specialties of medicine, but little general medicine.

Summary: Provides an easy way to study medicine for boards, but poor coverage. Average in the series.

Internal Medicine

$16.95   Review/test/221 q

Jarolim
Oklahoma Notes Series
Springer-Verlag 1993, 241 pages, ISBN 0-387-97960-3
Pros: Very quick reading in outline form. Covers most pertinent medical topics.
Cons: Looks like it was written on your grandparents' typewriter. Needs re-formatting. Questions provided are too simple with no explanations to the answers.
Summary: If you have limited time to study internal medicine, this may be the quickest way. But you won't get a good idea of typical board questions from this book. Best to supplement with other test questions.

Phantom Notes Medicine, 6th edition

$29.95   Review/0 q

Glickman
Phantom Notes Series
Phantom Notes 1992, 900 pages, ISBN 1-88093-400-0
Pros: Authors suggest to read this book five times, with the last reading completed within one day.
Cons: Outline form without enough detail in workup or treatment. Endless pages without interesting graphics.
Summary: Better books are available for boards review. Don't expect to have enough time or interest to read this dry outline repeatedly.

Specialty Board Review Internal Medicine, 3rd edition $39.95   Test/893 q

Pieroni
Specialty Board Review Series
Appleton & Lange 1990, 113 pages, ISBN 0-8385-8647-3
Pros: Good photographs.
Cons: Includes patient management problems (ie, which labs and studies to order) in a format not consistent with the USMLE, Step 2. Explanations are short and often explain the obvious, confirming what is already evident from the correct answer.
Summary: Not worth the big bucks.

NMS Introduction to Clinical Medicine, 1st edition $26.00   Review/test/300 q

Willms and Lewis
National Medical Series
Williams & Wilkins 1991, 260 pages, ISBN 0-683-06212-3
Pros: Provides review of history and physical exam skills.
Cons: Little applicability to boards. Material covered in this book can be easily learned through clinical experience.
Summary: Save your money—you don't need this one.

Harrison's Principles of Internal Medicine, 13th edition $98.00   Reference/0 q
Isselbacher et al
McGraw-Hill 1994, 2650 pages, ISBN 0-07-032370-4
Pros: Most complete medical textbook. Relatively many illustrations, graphs,
and x-ray images.
Cons: So densely written that it may be hard to read. Need to do extensive
searching to read complete details. Index needs improvement.
Summary: Your first choice for a standard medicine reference textbook.
Students going into any specialty should consider buying this classic.

 Internal Medicine, 4th edition $99.00   Reference/0 q
Stein
Mosby-Year Book 1994, 2861 + index, ISBN 0-8016-6911-1
Pros: Good coverage of basic physiology, use of diagnostic procedures
and tests, and specific diseases. Index is extensive.
Cons:
Summary: Very comprehensive textbook for more complete understanding
of disease. Highly recommended.

 Cecil Textbook of Medicine, 19th edition $92.85   Reference/0 q
Wyngaarden et al
Saunders 1992, 2536 pages, ISBN 0-7216-2928-8
Pros: Complete set of all the facts a medical student should know. Easier
to read than Harrison's. More cohesive because chapters are more
inclusive. Excellent index.
Cons: Fewer facts than Harrison's.
Summary: Although not as detailed as Harrison's, easier to read and
perhaps more useful to the time-limited medical student. Any further details
needed are best found in a primary source. Available in single and
two-volume sets.

 The Merck Manual, 16th edition $26.00   Reference/0 q
Merck
Merck 1992, 2844 pages, ISBN 0-911910-16-6
Pros: While not as comprehensive as either Cecil's or Harrison's bigger
volumes, this compact book is filled with enough information to provide
most fine points on almost any subject. Tabbed by subject and well
laid-out; topics are dealt with discretely so that there is little need for
index-rifling to gather all the facts. A good buy for the amount of information
given.
Cons: This book is billed as a "pocketbook" even though there's no way it
would fit in a pocket. It sacrifices tables, illustrations, and image-
reproductions for facts.
Summary: Perfect book for those on a budget who are not dependent on
graphics for their learning. Excellent for rapid learning of topic highlights.

Cecil Essentials of Medicine, 3rd edition $39.35   Reference

Andreoli

Saunders 1993, 921 pages, ISBN 0-7216-3272-6

Pros: Concise for quick reference. Good for understanding of physiology
and pathophysiology. Good tables.

Cons: Not good for quick reference of differential diagnosis or treatment.

Summary: Appropriate reference book for medical students. Cheaper than
other reference books.

B **Color Atlas and Text of Clinical Medicine** $39.95   Reference/0 q

Forbes

Mosby 1993, 521 pages, ISBN 0-8151-3271-9

Pros: Concise description of signs, symptoms, and evaluation, followed by
presentation of common and rare related disorders. 1433 excellent color
pictures and imaging, illustrating clinical signs of most major medical
disorders.

Cons: Can't be used as sole text.

Summary: Excellent for medical student as an illustrative introduction to
clinical medicine. Can be used with any of the major textbooks of medicine.

B **Essential Internal Medicine** $36.95   Reference/0 q

Kelley

Lippincott 1994, 826 pages, ISBN 0-397-51272-4

Pros: A soft-cover book that utilizes tables effectively and reaches enough
depth for day-to-day reading. Many good chapters on how various patient
presentations should be managed.

Cons: Simply not big enough to include all of the fine points of each
disease.

Summary: A mid-sized reference book, great for familiarizing yourself with
diseases, but a more comprehensive text is necessary to get all the fine
points on your patients' maladies. As usual in volumes of this size, there
are few illustrations or images.

B **Medicine for the Practicing Physician, 3rd edition** $125.00   Reference/0 q

Hurst

Reed 1992, 1983 pages, ISBN 0-7506-9072-0

Format (ie, test, review, reference)

Pros: Very discreet encapsulations. Chapters are inclusive, thus no need to
go index-searching. Clearly written.

Cons: Can't compete with Harrison's or Cecil's in terms of completeness.
Expensive. Very few graphics.

Summary: Great book for general review of various subjects, but not the
best reference available.

Internal Medicine Textbks

BOOK REVIEWS

B | **Textbook of Internal Medicine, 2nd edition** | $99.00 | Reference/0 q
Kelley
Lippincott 1992, 2441 pages + 182-page index, ISBN 0-397-51048-9
Pros: Large reference textbook, available to two volumes. Provides general pathophysiology, details of particular diseases, and approaches to diagnosis and management. Better in pathophysiology.
Cons: Poor in coverage of management. Could use more visual aids.
Summary: An alternative to consider buying as your "standard" reference textbook.

B | **The Principles and Practice of Medicine, 22nd edition** | $65.00 | Reference/0 q
Harvey et al
Appleton & Lange 1988, 1277 pages, ISBN 0-8385-7944-2
Pros: Among the major textbooks, best addresses pathophysiology and understanding of diseases.
Cons: Dry reading.
Summary: Directed toward medical students for a link between the basic and clinical sciences, but less useful for a practicing physician.

B− | **Internal Medicine Pearls** | $37.00 | Reference/0 q
Marsh
Pearls Series
Hanley & Belfus 1993, 276 pages, ISBN 1-56053-024-3
Pros: 100 case presentations, asking for diagnosis and treatment. Gives "pearls" to cover common problems. Glossy pages with good photos.
Cons: Cases are longer than would be seen on boards.
Summary: Probably not useful as reference on wards, but helpful in gaining diagnostic skills. Can be used for boards study, but involves a great deal of reading for limited "pearls" of wisdom.

B− | **Medical Secrets** | $35.95 | Reference/0 q
Zollo
Secrets Series
Hanley & Belfus 1991, 558 pages, ISBN 1-56053-011-1
Pros: Facts are presented as if in answer to a question, so it is fun to read along and see what is included in the responses. For that spare moment, provides a quick way to pick up a fact that will be interesting, if not always useful. Some very nice tables.
Cons: Really neither a handbook, review book, nor reference book. Supposedly used to answer "pimping" sessions. Some of the facts are trivial, and some of the answers you will have known already. An extra book to buy.
Summary: An interesting and thought-provoking book if you can afford something extra just for "fun." Not to be thought of as a replacement for a reference book or a boards preparation book.

C **Medicine, 3rd edition** $37.50   Reference/0 q

Fishman

Lippincott 1991, 555 pages, ISBN 0-397-51028-4

Pros: Clearly written, concise overview of medical topics. Good use of tables.

Cons: Too brief to contain the fine points of all medical subjects. Expensive for the amount of material it covers. Only illustrations are a few scattered x-rays.

Summary: Easy read but simply not complete enough, even for medical students.

Obstetrics and Gynecology On Call

$18.00 Handbook/0 q

Horowitz and Gomella
On Call Series
Appleton & Lange 1993, 640 pages, ISBN 0-8385-7174-3
Pros: Topics well-organized with discussions based around clinical
scenarios. Reviews pertinent questions and explains each step of
management.
Cons: Minimal illustrations. Not enough room for exhaustive discussions of
each topic.
Summary: Excellent organization for students on Ob-Gyn rotation but will
require a textbook companion if you are going into Ob-Gyn.

Handbook of Gynecology & Obstetrics

$24.95 Handbook/0 q

Brown and Crombleholme
Clinical Handbook Series
Appleton & Lange 1993, 546 pages, ISBN 0-8385-3608-5
Pros: Clear, concise, and organized with the most useful figures.
Pocket-sized.
Cons: Less information than *The Handbook of Obstetrics and Gynecology*
(but this might be a plus, depending on your perspective). Small print.
Summary: A smaller, truly pocket-sized handbook that gives up some
information but keeps the most important facts.

Handbook of Obstetrics and Gynecology, 9th edition

$29.00 Handbook/0 q

Benson and Pernoll
McGraw-Hill 1994, 817 pages, ISBN 0-07-105405-7
Pros: Very complete source in handbook size to take on wards. Useful
illustrations and extensive tables. Will be useful into residency.
Cons: Writing style is dense, making for slow reading in parts. Small print.
A bit thick and heavy to carry in a coat pocket.
Summary: A cheap yet thorough textbook in handbook size.

B+ **Manual of Clinical Problems in Obstetrics and Gynecology, 4th edition** $29.95   Handbook/0 q

Rivlin and Martin
Spiral Manual Series
Little, Brown 1994, 504 pages, ISBN 0-316-74777-7
Pros: Concise narrative divided into topics. Five to 10 minutes of reading gives an overview of all the most pertinent facts.
Cons: Material extremely dense, sometimes requiring deciphering of passages. Lack of space causes some loss of background discussions. No graphs or figures.
Summary: Great reference tool for the wards or boning-up on subjects for the boards, but will have to be supplemented for more than barest knowledge of these subjects.

A

Appleton & Lange's Review of Obstetrics & Gynecology, 5th edition

$25.95   Test/1600+ q

Julian et al

Appleton & Lange Review Series

Appleton & Lange 1995, 397 pages, ISBN 0-8385-0231-8

Pros: Comprehensive review of Ob-Gyn through multiple-choice questions and excellent anatomical drawings. Good sections on diseases during pregnancy and primary health care for women, both topics covered on boards but not found in many boards review books.

Cons: Some topics, such as surgical technique, are not useful for USMLE Step 2. Moderately expensive.

Summary: Excellent questions and explanations. A very good review for those who need to emphasize their studying on Ob-Gyn.

B

NMS Obstetrics and Gynecology, 3rd edition

$28.00   Review/test/500 q

Beck, Jr.

National Medical Series

Williams & Wilkins 1993, 484 pages, ISBN 0-683-06241-7

Pros: Detailed review of obstetrics and gynecology in extended outline form. Includes study questions at the end of each section, plus a comprehensive exam. The comprehensive exam includes good clinical scenarios.

Cons: Too long for Step 2 review. Older editions are shorter.

Summary: Average among the NMS series. Consider using an older edition if you want a quicker review.

B

Obstetrics and Gynecology

$16.95   Review/104 q

Miles et al

Oklahoma Notes Series

Springer-Verlag 1994, 226 pages, ISBN 0-387-94184-3

Pros: Easy-to-read outline format. Coverage of both normal and abnormal obstetrics. Good for rapid review of major topics. Many excellent charts, plus a few good illustrations.

Cons: Sometimes lacks necessary details, particularly on management.

Summary: Average among the Oklahoma Notes series.

PreTest Obstetrics and Gynecology, 7th edition

B

$16.95   Test/500 q

Evans

PreTest Self-Assessment and Review Series

McGraw-Hill 1995, 231 pages, ISBN 0-07-0520267

Pros: Some improvement over last edition by deleting some sections. Concise answers.

Cons: Still contains type-K questions. Good learning material, but most questions are shorter and less clinically oriented than boards-style questions. Sections are too short to comprehensively cover Ob-Gyn.

Summary: Average among the PreTest series. Not comprehensive enough.

Comprehensive Gynecology Review, 2nd edition

B⁻

$25.95   Test/900 q

Holzman et al

Mosby-Year Book 1992, 298 pages, ISBN 0-8016-2279-4

Pros: This is a companion test book for the textbook, *Comprehensive Gynecology,* by Arthur L. Herbst et al. Topics are arranged in accord with chapters from the textbook. Covers basic gynecology with good explanations.

Cons: Does not include obstetrics. Includes some controversial topics which would not be used on standard exams. Many K-type questions.

Summary: Comprehensive coverage of gynecology, but does not include obstetrics. Excellent questions and explanations, but too expensive to cover only a portion of the Step 2 exam.

Obstetrics & Gynecology Review 1994, 8th edition

C

$45.00   Review/test/284 q

Sheld

McGraw-Hill 1994, 565 pages, ISBN 0-07-056442-6

Pros: Answers are clearly referenced to recent articles from the *American Journal of Obstetrics and Gynecology* and *Obstetrics and Gynecology.* Very up-to-date.

Cons: Answers are too long and detailed. Too expensive.

Summary: Not suited to boards review for medical students.

Ob-Gyn Review Books

BOOK REVIEWS

104

Danforth's Obstetrics and Gynecology, 7th edition $125.00   Reference/0 q
Scott et al
Lippincott 1994, 1121 pages, ISBN 0-397-51353-4
Pros: Comprehensive textbook of both obstetrics and gynecology.
Well-organized and easy to read.
Cons: Expensive.
Summary: An excellent resource, but for medical students not considering a
career in Ob-Gyn, this book is too detailed and too expensive.

 Williams Obstetrics, 19th edition $95.00   Reference/0 q
Cunningham et al
Appleton & Lange 1993, 1428 pages, ISBN 0-8385-9634-7
Pros: Comprehensive textbook of obstetrics. Appropriate use of line
drawings and photos.
Cons: Does not include gynecology.
Summary: Not needed for an Ob-Gyn rotation, but is an excellent resource
for the future obstetrician.

 Basic Gynecology and Obstetrics, $34.95   Reference/0 q
Gant et al
Appleton & Lange 1993, 472 pages, ISBN 0-8385-9633-9
Pros: Well-written, well-illustrated textbook with in-depth information
sufficient for the wards.
Cons:
Summary: Moderately priced textbook for third-year students who want to
be well-informed for wards, but too long for a review book and not
in-depth enough for residency.

 Essentials of Obstetrics and Gynecology, 2nd edition $34.65   Reference/0 q
Hacker and Moore
Saunders 1992, 634 pages, ISBN 10-7216-3668-3
Pros: Complete Ob text complete with tables, figures, and relatively in-depth
treatment of these topics. Easy-to-read writing style with easy-on-the-eyes
print.
Cons: Some depth traded off for clarity and larger print.
Summary: Coverage of subjects is more than adequate for medical students
but text lacks versatility; neither concise enough for board study nor
complete enough to be a reference for those going into Ob-Gyn.

Obstetrics and Gynecology for Medical Students

$33.00   Reference/0 q

Beckman et al

Williams & Wilkins 1992, 427 pages, ISBN 0-683-0500-6

Pros: A manageable book for busy medical students. Encapsulates major topics and presents them in easy-to-digest manner. Provides set of objectives for students to learn. Scarce but good use of graphics. Review questions are relatively few but include explanations.

Cons: Not overly ambitious. Subjects tend to be presented simplistically and topics tend to be treated in the most basic way.

Summary: Could be the text of choice for students looking to "survive" the Ob-Gyn rotation. Easy-to-read and well-written but information often sketchy. Reading select chapters may be moderately useful for boards review.

Current Obstetric & Gynecologic Diagnosis and Treatment, 8th edition

$41.95   Reference/0 q

DeCherney and Pernoll

Current Series

Appleton & Lange 1994, 1227 pages, ISBN 0-8385-1447-2

Pros: Softcover reference text with many diagrams, anatomical drawings, black and white photos. Good coverage, adequate for medical students.

Cons: Although information provided is good, does not facilitiate differential diagnosis. Expensive for medical students.

Summary: Cheaper alternatives available for a medical student. Standard texts should first be considered for potential Ob-Gyn residents.

Obstetrical Pearls, 2nd edition

$16.95   Reference/0 q

Benson

Davis 1994, 214 pages, ISBN 0-8036-0702-4

Pros: Practical clinical guide to obstetrics, including some procedural information. Rapid reading of the entire text within a few hours. Pocket-sized.

Cons: Oriented to clinical, does not always emphasize non-clinical facts. An overview, therefore, somewhat sketchy. Does not include gynecology.

Summary: May be useful as a "down and dirty" source of facts to review before starting an Ob rotation, but not complete enough for a rotation exam or boards review. Too basic to be useful to a resident.

The Harriet Lane Handbook, 13th edition

$25.95   Handbook/0 q

Johnson

Mosby-Yearbook 1993, 658 pages, ISBN 0-8016-8000-X

Pros: This is the peds equivalent of the Scut Monkey Handbook. Includes most common pediatric drugs and dosages, as well as excellent information on pediatric emergency management and diagnostic tests. Pocket sized.

Cons: Expensive investment if you do not plan to stay in pediatrics.

Summary: A "must-have" on the pediatric rotation. If you will only be doing one pediatrics rotation and have no future plans to treat children, then borrow this one.

Pediatric Pearls—The Handbook of Practical Pediatrics, 2nd edition

$30.00   Handbook/0 q

Rosenstein et al

Year Book Handbooks

Mosby-Year Book 1993, 368 pages, ISBN 0-8016-7171-X

Pros: Brief descriptions of problems and conditions, plus recommendations for treatment and management. Organized by organ systems. This is presented in an easy-to-read and practical manner. Pocket-sized.

Cons: Not many tables or illustrations. A better reference book might be needed during the peds rotation. Expensive.

Summary: Excellent reference for medical management of most common conditions. Good companion to *The Harriet Lane Handbook.*

B   Handbook of Pediatrics, 17th edition,

$27.00   Handbook/0 q

Merenstein et al

Appleton & Lange 1994, 1071 pages, ISBN 0-8385-3657-3

Pros: Concise descriptions of diseases and treatment. Good tables.

Cons: Too thick and heavy to carry in your pocket.

Summary: Good reference book for the pediatric clerkship, but since it's too thick to carry in your white coat pocket, consider investing in a better softcover reference text.

Manual of Pediatric Therapeutics, 5th edition

$28.50   Handbook/0 q

Graef

Little, Brown 1994, 691 pages, ISBN 0-316-13875-4

Pros: Concise outline format, providing general principles, management, and treatment of most common diseases and conditions in pediatrics. Good tables and charts. Good size to carry in a large white coat pocket.

Cons: Neglects some specific conditions that might be seen in a tertiary care center.

Summary: Good comprehensive manual for third-year pediatric clerkship and for quick reference as a pediatric resident.

Appleton & Lange's Review of Pediatrics, 5th edition

$26.95   Test/1000+ q

Lorin
Appleton & Lange Review Series
Appleton & Lange 1993, 222 pages, ISBN 0-8385-0057-9
Pros: Has a "warm-up" question section that teaches exam-taking skills.
Excellent coverage of the most important pediatric topics covered on the
boards, including development and accidents. Answers are short and
concise.
Cons: Questions generally tend to be shorter than Step 2 questions.
However, there is a case management section that includes longer
clinical scenarios and a series of questions, more indicative of boards-style
questions.
Summary: Expensive, but has comprehensive coverage for those who need
a better review of pediatrics.

NMS Pediatrics, 2nd edition

$28.00   Test/review/475 q

Dworkin
National Medical Series
Harwal 1992, 550 pages, ISBN 0-683-06246-8
Pros: Outline format useful for rotation and boards review. Provides
comprehensive coverage.
Cons: Too long for Step 2 review, but useful for a boards-style rotation
exam. Not as good for learning as softcover textbooks.
Summary: Above average for NMS series.

Pediatrics

$16.95   Review/50 q

Osburn
Oklahoma Notes Series
Springer-Verlag 1993, 257 pages, ISBN 0-387-97955-7, 3-540-97955-7
Pros: Brief coverage of major topics. Many useful charts. Several chapters
open with helpful facts on developmental issues. Some chapters also have
brief disease profiles, covering etiology, pathophysiology, physical and
laboratory findings, and therapy. One of the better books in the Oklahoma
Notes series.
Cons: Chapters written by several authors, thus quality varies. Generally
easy to read, but several different formats used. At times, covers
information helpful for your general knowledge but which is not testable
material. Short practice test is not representative of boards material. Typos
throughout the book can be misleading, particularly for abbreviations.
Summary: This will provide the quickest review of pediatrics available for
Step 2. The quality of the material varies throughout the book, but is
generally helpful.

B | **PreTest Pediatrics, 7th edition** | **$16.95** | Test/500 q

Schaeffer et al
PreTest Series
McGraw-Hill 1995, 250 pages, ISBN 0-07-052027-5
Pros: Good section on general pediatrics which emphasizes behavior and development. Includes questions on what is "normal," a heavily stessed topic on boards. Has good balance of both factual questions and case scenarios.
Cons: New editions contain many identical questions from previous editions.
Summary: A good buy, but if you can borrow an old edition, it's even better!

B⁻ | **Pediatrics, 9th edition** | **$26.95** | Test/700 q

Hansbarger
MEPC Series
Appleton & Lange 1995, 248 pages, ISBN 0-8385-6223-X
Pros: Offers a large number of questions for review.
Cons: Depth and complexity of questions are not up to the level of the USMLE Step 2. Includes old K-type questions.
Summary: This should not be a first-line choice for pediatrics test review.

Fundamentals of Pediatrics

$37.95   Reference/0 q

Rudolph et al

Appleton & Lange 1994, 701 pages, ISBN 0-8385-8233-8

Pros: Information presented in a very concise and organized manner.
Multiple algorithms show approaches to the evaluation, diagnosis, and
management of common conditions. Easy to read.

Cons: A more complete text needed if you're considering a pediatric residency.

Summary: Good reference book for pediatric clerkship and for your library
if you are considering primary care or pediatrics.

Principles and Practice of Pediatrics, 2nd edition

$99.50   Reference/0 q

Oski

Lippincott 1994, 2368 pages, ISBN 0-397-51221-X

Pros: Good explanations of epidemiology and pathogenesis. Clinical
manifestations, diagnosis, and treatment also well-addressed. Includes 29
interesting color pictures, plus many more black and white photos. Best use
of graphics among major pediatric reference books.

Cons:

Summary: Excellent pediatric reference text, particularly for those
considering primary care or pediatrics.

Nelson Essentials of Pediatrics, 2nd edition

$36.50   Reference/0 q

Behrman et al

Saunders 1994, 795 pages, ISBN 0-7216-3775-2

Pros: Faster and easier to read than its parent hardcover reference book.

Cons: Dry reading.

Summary: Provides sufficient information to give a basic understanding of
pediatric problems.

Nelson Textbook of Pediatrics, 14th edition

$91.40   Reference/0 q

Behrman

Saunders 1992, 1965 pages, ISBN 0-7216-2976-8

Pros: Considered by many as the standard pediatrics textbook.

Cons: Slow reading. Fewer photos.

Summary: An excellent pediatric reference text, but should not be bought
by a medical student unless you will be doing primary care or pediatrics.

Current Pediatric Diagnosis and Treatment, 12th edition

$41.95   Reference/0 q

Hay, Jr. et al
Current Series
Appleton & Lange 1995, 1295 pages, ISBN 0-8385-1446-4
Pros: Better soft-cover textbook than the "baby" editions of the major hardcovers. Use of some algorithms.
Cons: Expensive. Less detailed on treatment.
Summary: A soft-cover textbook to use as an alternative to the major hardcover textbooks.

Pediatric Medicine, 2nd edition

$99.00   Reference/0 q

Avery and First
Williams & Wilkins 1994, 1636 pages, ISBN 0-683-00293-7
Pros: Easier reading than other major pediatric textbooks, but not as detailed with shorter chapters. Interesting use of case illustrations with accompanying question and comment.
Cons:
Summary: Good option.

Pediatric Secrets

$33.95   Reference/0 q

Polin et al
Secrets Series
Hanley & Belfus Inc. 1989, 447 pages, ISBN 0-932883-14-1
Pros: Question-and-answer format is east to read. Numerous curious facts invite you to continue with the reading. Contains details to impress your attending.
Cons: Does not present a broad discussion of any topic in specific. A second reference book for details is needed.
Summary: Excellent book to read when you do not feel like studying.

Rudolph's Pediatrics, 19th edition

$95.00   Reference/0 q

Rudolph
Appleton & Lange 1991, 2111 pages, ISBN 0-8385-8488-8
Pros: Very comprenhensive textbook of pediatrics.
Cons: Oldest edition among the major pediatric textbooks. The softcover "baby" edition is more useful for a pediatrics rotation, particularly for those not choosing this field as a career.
Summary: Another hardcover pediatric reference textbook to consider for those entering primary care or pediatrics residencies.

PreTest Preventive Medicine and Public Health, 7th edition

$16.95 Test/500 q

Scutchfield

PreTest Self-Assessment and Review Series

McGraw-Hill 1995, 213 pages, ISBN 0-07-052066-6

Pros: Good sections on biostatistics, epidemiology, and preventive medicine. Studying these questions and answers will provide an adequate review for Step 2.

Cons: Sections on health services and legal and ethical issues are less useful.

Summary: One of the better PreTest books. If you prefer to learn by the question and answer method, this is the best available book on preventive medicine and public health.

NMS Preventive Medicine and Public Health, 2nd edition

$27.00 Review/450 q

Cassens

National Medical Series

Harwal 1992, 497 pages, ISBN 0-683-06262-X

Pros: The most comprehensive preventive medicine and public health review book designed for Step 2 use.

Cons: Simply too long with a relatively low yield.

Summary: Poor investment of time and money.

NMS Clinical Epidemiology and Biostatistics

$29.00 Review/test/300 q

Knapp and Miller III

National Medical Series

Williams & Wilkins 1992, 435 pages, ISBN 0-683-06206-9

Pros: Detailed coverage of statistics.

Cons: Simply too long for boards review.

Summary: Most students will find this to be overkill for boards review of statistics.

Behavioral Sciences, 4th edition

$17.95 Review/169 q

Krug and Cass

Oklahoma Notes Series

Springer-Verlag 1995, 311 pages, ISBN 0-387-94393-5

Pros: Outline format allows for rapid reading. Includes quite a bit on psychiatry.

Cons: Designed for Step 1. Does not include preventive medicine. Section on health care systems is the only part of the book that addresses public health.

Summary: Designed for Step 1 and therefore not very helpful for Step 2 review. If you already own this text, it could be used for psychiatry review, but better sources are available.

BOOK REVIEWS

Preventive Medicine

Psychiatry Handbooks

begin on page 115

Psychiatry, 5th edition

$22.95   Handbook/0 q

Tomb
House Officer Series
Williams & Wilkins 1995, 292 pages, ISBN 0-683-08343-0
Pros: Excellent handbook, but also will serve as a very useful boards
review. Summaries are brief but highlight important points. Section on
biological therapy is important for boards study. New edition based on
DSM-IV.
Cons: None.
Summary: This is an excellent investment for both a psychiatry rotation and
for boards review.

The Handbook of Psychiatry

$31.95   Handbook/0 q

Residents of the UCLA Department of Psychiatry; Guze
Year Book Handbook Series
Year Book 1990, 727 pages, ISBN 0-8151-3644-7
Pros: Detailed coverage of psychiatry. More extensive coverage of
psychotherapy than other handbooks. Also has good pharmacotherapy
coverage.
Cons: Could be used for boards review, but more detailed than needed for
that purpose.
Summary: A good handbook that can be used for a psychiatry rotation or for
boards review.

Pocket Handbook of Clinical Psychiatry

$32.00   Handbook/0 q

Kaplan and Sadock
Williams & Wilkins 1990, 335 pages, ISBN 0-683-04523-7
Pros: First chapter includes a rapid review of major psychiatric disorders in
just seven pages. Good use of tables, including diagnostic criteria.
Cons: Based on DSM-III-R. Not pocket-sized.
Summary: A good handbook that can be used for a psychiatry rotation or
for boards review.

Psychiatry, 2nd edition

$7.75   Handbook/0 q

Burwell and Cucciarella
Current Clinical Strategies
CCS Publishing 1995, 96 pages, ISBN 1-881528-14-6
Pros: Small enough to fit in pants pocket.
Cons: Incomplete of description of psychiatric disorders by diagnostic
criteria and mental status examination findings.
Summary: Simply not complete enough to be useful. Drug information can
be found in any standard medicine handbook.

BOOK REVIEWS

Psychiatry Handbooks

Psychiatry Review Books

begin on page 117

PreTest Psychiatry, 7th edition

$16.95   Test/500 q

Woods
PreTest Series
McGraw-Hill 1995, 213 pages, ISBN 0-07-052064-X
Pros: Well-written answers cover important boards material.
Cons: Includes K-type questions.
Summary: One of the better books in the PreTest series. Good review of psychiatry.

NMS Psychiatry, 2nd edition

$28.00   Test/review/500 q

Scully et al
National Medical Series
Williams & Wilkins 1990, 335 pages, ISBN 0-683-06264-6
Pros: Detailed outline form. Complete coverage makes this book useful for both rotation and boards study.
Cons: Somewhat too long for Step 2 review.
Summary: Comprehensive coverage of psychiatry but too long for most medical students to complete for Step 2 review. Valuable as a rotation reference book or for selected study in weak areas.

B Appleton & Lange's Review of Psychiatry, 5th edition

$26.95   Test/900+ q

Easson
Appleton & Lange's Review Series
Appleton & Lange 1994, 178 pages, ISBN 0-8385-0247-4
Pros: Question and answer format divided by topics. Also has extra sections of matching-set questions, one-best-answer questions, case histories, and a practice test. Gives diagnostic nomenclature for both DSM-III-R and DSM-IV.
Cons: Quality of explanations varies—brief but sometimes too basic without enough detail.
Summary: Large number of questions but still costly for Step 2 review. Do not expect to see emphasis of changes in DSM-IV on Step 2.

B Psychiatry, 10th edition

$16.95   Test/700 q

Chan and Prosen
Medical Exam Review Series
Appleton & Lange 1995, 257 pages, ISBN 0-8385-5780-5
Pros: Good coverage of basic psychiatry material. Short questions and explanations allow for a relatively rapid review of psychiatry.
Cons: Explanations generally short, providing little in-depth information.
Summary: Above average among the Medical Exam Review series.

B Study Guide and Self-Examination Review for Kaplan and Sadock's Synopsis of Psychiatry, 5th edition

$45.00   Test/review/ 1000+ q

Kaplan and Sadock
Williams & Wilkins 1994, 482 pages, ISBN 0-683-04541-5
Pros: Keyed to the seventh edition of *Kaplan and Sadock's Synopsis of Psychiatry*. Each chapter contains an introduction, a list of key terms and concepts, and boards-type questions. Questions address most important topics, and answers give complete explanations. All terms and conditions are consistent with DSM-IV.
Cons: Chapter introductions cover important basics, but details of the key terms and concepts are not included. Includes K-type questions. Very expensive.
Summary: Excellent study guide for those interested in psychiatry. High-yield questions and answers, but too expensive for a boards budget.

C Psychiatry

$16.95   Review/0 q

Shaffer and Krug
Oklahoma Notes Series
Springer-Verlag 1993, 188 pages, ISBN 0-387-97957-3, 3-540-97957-3
Pros: Outline form. Rapid reading.
Cons: Not enough detail. Includes too much low-yield information.
Summary: Better suited toward rapid review for a psychiatry rotation than for boards review.

Clinical Psychiatry for Medical Students, 2nd edition $37.50 Reference/0 q

Stoudemire

Lippincott 1994, 717 pages, ISBN 0-397-51338-0

Pros: Clear writing style and good layout make this easy to read. Case vignettes are illustrative.

Cons: Does not specifically list DSM-IV diagnostic criteria, but does give good adaptations that give important highlights.

Summary: Excellent psychiatry text for reference. Too long for boards review.

Review of General Psychiatry, 4th edition $32.95 Reference/0 q

Goldman

Appleton & Lange 1995, 535 pages, ISBN 0-8385-8421-7

Pros: Good coverage, including treatment. Short tables are clear, emphasize salient points, and show useful comparisons. Based on DSM-IV.

Cons: Could improve differential diagnosis.

Summary: Excellent text for rotation study. Too long for boards review.

B Kaplan and Sadock's Synopsis of Psychiatry, 7th edition $55.00 Reference/0 q

Kaplan et al

Williams & Wilkins 1994, 1257 pages, ISBN 0-683-04530-X

Pros: Written by the authors of the "gold standard" in psychiatry, *Comprehensive Textbook of Psychiatry*. One of the most comprehensive soft-cover psych books. Good glossaries of terms and excellent use of tables.

Cons: Expensive and too long for most medical students.

Summary: Terrific for medical students interested in psychiatry residency. Otherwise, cost and length are prohibitive for most.

B Psychiatry for Medical Students, 2nd edition $38.50 Reference/0 q

Waldinger

American Psychiatric Press, 615 pages, ISBN 0-88048-373-3

Pros: Very easy and quick reading. Generally good explanations of differential diagnosis. Good tables using diagnostic criteria.

Cons: Needs up-dating. Based on DSM-III-R. Sometimes wordy.

Summary: An average psychiatry text for medical students. Not adequate for psychiatry residency. Too lengthy for boards review.

BOOK REVIEWS

Psychiatry Textbooks

C Psychiatric Diagnosis, 4th edition $19.95   Reference/0 q

Goodwin and Guze

Oxford University Press 1989, 332 pages, ISBN 0-19-505231-5

Pros: Softcover reference text with more attention to "how" and "why" by citing results of studies.

Cons: Out-of-date. Does not cover recently developed psychiatric drugs, often uses older terminology, and neglects most personality disorders.

Summary: Poor investment. Many better texts and handbooks are available.

The Surgical Intern Pocket Survival Guide, 2nd edition   **$6.00**   Handbook/0 q

Chamberlain
Intern Pocket Survival Guide Series
International Medical Publishing 1993, 74 pages, ISBN 0-9634063-5-3
Pros: Very practical coverage of medical management of surgical patients.
Examples of orders are helpful for new medical students. Plenty of
information for the price of a movie.
Cons: None.
Summary: Useful to carry around at all times on the surgery wards. A wise
investment.

 Handbook of Surgery, 10th edition,   **$30.00**   Handbook/0 q

Schrock
Yearbook Handbook Series
Mosby 1994, 1013 pages, ISBN 0-8016-7637-1
Pros: More comprehensive than other handbooks.
Cons: Less detailed on treatment than other handbooks. Slightly too thick to
fit in most white coat pockets.
Summary: A good investment for the surgery rotation. Could be used for
rapid review of surgery for the boards.

 Manual of Surgical Therapeutics, 8th edition   **$30.00**   Handbook/0 q

Condon and Nyhus
Little, Brown Spiral Manual Series
Little, Brown 1993, 418 pages, ISBN 0-316-15367-2
Pros: Format similar to that of *The Washington Manual.* Very practical and
pertinent to the surgical patient.
Cons: Too large to carry around in a pocket. Expensive for a handbook.
Summary: Helpful handbook. If you have the money, it's worth the
investment.

 Principles of Surgery Companion Handbook, 6th edition   **$27.50**   Handbook/0 q

Schwartz
McGraw-Hill 1994, 771 pages, ISBN 0-07-056055-2
Pros: Concise reference, based on one of the most popular surgery
textbooks. Includes pathophysiology and general treatment.
Cons: Heavy handbook that serves as a good reference, but less practical
for rounds and orders.
Summary: Good buy, especially if you're interested in surgery.

Surgery On Call, 2nd edition

$21.95   Handbook/0 q

Gomella and Lefor
On Call Series
Appleton & Lange 1990, 436 pages, ISBN 0-8385-8738-0
Pros: Covers many problems seen while on call. Includes questions you
should ask yourself.
Cons: Many problems are the same as seen in Medicine. Lab interpretation
and commonly used medications section is similar to that seen in the
Scut Monkey Handbook.
Summary: Good pocketbook for medical students but not complete enough.

A⁻ NMS Surgery, 2nd edition

$28.00   Test/review/418 q

Jarell and Carabasi III
National Medical Series
Harwal Publishing 1991, 556 pages, ISBN 0-683-06270-0
Pros: Good review for boards. Outline format followed by study questions.
Questions presented as clinical cases.
Cons: Study questions, although they follow USMLE format, are too simple.
Summary: Provides an excellent review in a logical and well-organized
manner, even though the study questions do not match the level of difficulty
of the USMLE. Helpful for rotation exam.

B PreTest Surgery, 7th edition

$16.95   Test/261 q

King, Geller, Chabot
PreTest Series
McGraw-Hill 1992, 261 pages, ISBN 0-07-052013-5
Pros: In-depth questions that will test many aspects of your knowledge
about surgery. Also tests subspecialties. Answers generally provide
concise, lucid review.
Cons: Questions do not reflect those on the USMLE—often either too
difficult or too simple. Includes old K-type questions.
Summary: Not reflective of material stressed on the USMLE, but useful as
a review of surgery. For the price, not a bad buy for review while on the
surgery rotation.

B Surgery, 2nd edition

$29.95   Review/0 q

Glickman, Jr. et al
Phantom Notes Series
Phantom Notes 1992, 541 pages, ISBN 1-880934-01-9
Pros: Pocket-sized, so good to carry on the wards for quick review of any
topic. Outline form covers most pertinent facts. Good descriptions of
surgical treatment *and* reasons for these treatments.
Cons: Too extensive for a *quick* review the night before an exam. No
diagrams or illustrations.
Summary: Clear and well-written. If outline format appeals to you, this may
well be your first choice.

B **Surgery, 11th edition** $16.95   Test/700 q

Metzler
Medical Exam Review Series
Appleton & Lange 1995, 317 pages, ISBN 0-8385-6195-0
Pros: Good variety of questions. Includes quality pictures. Oddly contains a
chapter on statistics and clinical literature interpretation, not relevant to
surgery, but illustrative of important terms for boards review.
Cons: Covers too many surgical subspecialties and not enough general
surgery.
Summary: Average among Medical Exam Review series.

B⁻ **General Surgery** $16.95   Review/0 q

Jacocks
Oklahoma Notes Series
Springer-Verlag 1993, 142 pages, ISBN 0-387-97958-1, 3-540-97958-1
Pros: Organized by organ systems. Addresses common clinical problems
and differential diagnoses. Outline format with important facts allows for
quick and easy review.
Cons: Not very much detail, often too simplified. No practice test questions.
Summary: Good for quick review, but too simplified.

D **Principles of Surgery Self Assessment and Review,** $39.95   Test/review/600 q
6th edition

Schwartz
McGraw-Hill 1994, 228 pages, ISBN 0-07-052012-7
Pros:
Cons: Designed for residents preparing for the American Board of Surgery
Qualifying, In-Training, and Certifying Examinations and for board-certified
surgeons preparing for recertification. The questions are too difficult to be
used as a review for the USMLE Step 2.
Summary: Too difficult.

Essentials of General Surgery, 2nd edition

$35.00   Reference/187 q

Lawrence
Essentials Series
Williams & Wilkins 1992, 432 pages, ISBN 0-683-04869-4
Pros: Well-written with good photos. Illustrations cover most pertinent
anatomy. Designed for medical students.
Cons: Does not include boards-style questions.
Summary: Excellent choice as an introductory textbook for medical
students.

Principles of Surgery, 6th edition

$99.00   Reference/0 q

Schwartz
McGraw-Hill 1994, 2183 pages, ISBN 0-07-055928-7
Pros: Well-written, the most complete textbook. Figures of all types are
used liberally.
Cons: Small print.
Summary: An up-to-date fully referenced text that must be considered by
those going into surgery.

Textbook of Surgery, 14th edition

$89.10   Reference/0 q

Sabiston, Jr.
Saunders 1991, 2208 pages, ISBN 0-7216-3492-3
Pros: Well-written, well-illustrated, complete surgical reference book with
exhaustive index. Gives historical data as well as the purely "useful" data.
Cons: Too extensive for most medical students.
Summary: One of the definitive texts for those going into surgery.

Current Surgical Diagnosis and Treatment, 10th edition $41.95   Reference/0 q

Way
Current Series
Appleton & Lange 1994, 1341 pages, ISBN 0-8385-1439-1
Pros: Excellent book for the medical students as a reference and textbook.
Brief and concise descriptions of diseases followed by diagnosis and
treatment (or current management). Easy to read and understand. Good
illustrations.
Cons:
Summary: Quick source of information for management of surgical diseases.
Good reference book for students, residents, and primary care physicians.

B⁻ **Lecture Notes on General Surgery, 8th edition**   **$29.95**   Reference/0 q

Ellis and Calmo
Lecture Notes Series
Blackwell Scientific 1993, 377 pages, ISBN 0-632-03335-5
Pros: Very concise. Contains the most important surgery facts in basic outline form.
Cons: Written in the U.K., therefore some terminology, as well as treatment, is different than in the U.S.
Summary: If outline formats appeal to you, this is a decent investment, but not a first choice.

B⁻ **Surgical Basic Science**   **$48.00**   Reference/0 q

Fischer
Mosby 1993, 524 pages, ISBN 0-8016-6441-1
Format (ie, test, review, reference)
Pros: Good reference for physiology and theory behind surgical practice.
Cons: Emphasis on physiology and pathophysiology results in little focus on patient management or any surgical procedures. Does not address anatomy. Not many illustrations.
Summary: More of a textbook than a reference book. Not practical, thus medical students would need another reference to manage patients. Not a good buy for a surgery clerkship book.

C **Basic Surgery, 4th edition**   **$40.00**   Reference/200 q

Polk et al
Quality Medical Publishing 1993, 884 pages, ISBN 0-942219-29-5
Pros: Covers everything. Includes crucial illustrations. Good index.
Cons: Long. Too much information. Not always clearly written.
Summary: Contains all the facts, but too many to be useful in boards review or for reference in the few hours available to the average medical student during a surgery rotation. But it is a complete text that might be useful to persons planning on a surgical residency.

Surgery Textbooks

BOOK REVIEWS

Book Index

Subject Index

Basic Science Textbooks

Biochemistry
Examination & Board Review
Balcavage & King
1995, ISBN 0-8385-0661-5, A0661-7

Color Atlas of Basic Histology
Berman
1993, ISBN 0-8385-0445-0, A0445-5

1996 First Aid for the USMLE Step 1
Bhushan, et al.
1996, ISBN 0-8385-2597-0, A2597-1

Jawetz, Melnick, & Adelberg's
Medical Microbiology, 20/e
Brooks, Butel, & Ornston
1995, ISBN 0-8385-6243-4, A6243-8

Manual for Human Dissection
Photographs with Clinical Applications
Callas
1994, ISBN 0-8385-6133-0, A6133-1

Concise Pathology, 2/e
Chandrasoma & Taylor
1995, ISBN 0-8385-1229-1, A1229-2

Introduction to Clinical Psychiatry
Elkin
1996, ISBN 0-8385-4333-2, A4333-9

Medical Biostatistics & Epidemiology
Examination & Board Review
Essex-Sorlie
1995, ISBN 0-8385-6219-1, A6219-8

**Fundamentals of Medical Cell Biology
and Histology**
Fuller
1996, ISBN 0-8385-1384-0, A1384-5

Review of Medical Physiology, 17/e
Ganong
1995, ISBN 0-8385-8431-4, A8431-7

First Aid for the USMLE Step 2
A Student-to-Student Guide
Go, Curet-Salim, & Fullerton
1996, ISBN 0-8385-2591-1, A2591-4

Medical Epidemiology, 2/e
Greenberg, Daniels, Flanders, Eley, & Boring
1996, ISBN 0-8385-6206-X, A6206-5

Basic Histology, 8/e
Junqueira, Carneiro, & Kelley
1995, ISBN 0-8385-0567-8, A0567-6

Basic & Clinical Pharmacology, 6/e
Katzung
1995, ISBN 0-8385-0619-4, A0619-5

Pharmacology
Examination & Board Review, 4/e
Katzung & Trevor
1995, ISBN 0-8385-8067-X, A8067-9

First Aid for the Match
Le, Bhushan, & Amin
1996, ISBN 0-8385-2596-2, A2596-3

Medical Microbiology & Immunology
Examination & Board Review, 4/e
Levinson & Jawetz
1996, ISBN 0-8385-6225-6, A6225-5

Clinical Anatomy
Lindner
1989, ISBN 0-8385-1259-3, A1259-9

Pathophysiology of Disease
McPhee, Lingappa, Ganong, & Lange
1995, ISBN 0-8385-7815-2, A7815-2

Harper's Biochemistry, 23/e
Murray, Granner, Mayes, & Rodwell
1993, ISBN 0-8385-3562-3, A3562-4

Pathology
Examination & Board Review
Newland
1995, ISBN 0-8385-7719-9, A7719-6

Basic Histology
Examination & Board Review, 3/e
Paulsen
1996, ISBN 0-8385-2282-3, A2282-0

Basic & Clinical Immunology, 8/e
Stites, Terr, & Parslow
1994, ISBN 0-8385-0561-9, A0561-9

Correlative Neuroanatomy, 22/e
Waxman & deGroot
1995, ISBN 0-8385-1091-4, A1091-6

Clinical Science Textbooks

Clinical Neurology, 3/e
Aminoff, Greenberg, & Simon
1996, ISBN 0-8385-1383-2, A1383-7

Understanding Health Policy:
A Clinical Approach
Bodenheimer & Grumbach
1995, ISBN 0-8385-3678-6, A3678-8

(more on reverse)

Clinical Cardiology, 6/e
Cheitlin, Sokolow, & McIlroy
1993, ISBN 0-8385-1093-0, A1093-2
Fluid & Electrolytes
Physiology & Pathophysiology
Cogan
1991, ISBN 0-8385-2546-6, A2546-8
Basic & Clinical Biostatistics, 2/e
Dawson-Saunders & Trapp
1994, ISBN 0-8385-0542-2, A0542-9
Basic Gynecology and Obstetrics
Gant & Cunningham
1993, ISBN 0-8385-9633-9, A9633-7
Review of General Psychiatry, 4/e
Goldman
1995, ISBN 0-8385-8421-7, A8421-8
Principles of Clinical Electrocardiography, 13/e
Goldschlager & Goldman
1990, ISBN 0-8385-7951-5, A7951-5
Basic & Clinical Endocrinology, 4/e
Greenspan & Baxter
1994, ISBN 0-8385-0560-0, A0560-1
Occupational Medicine
LaDou
1990, ISBN 0-8385-7207-3, A7207-2
Primary Care of Women
Lemcke, Pattison, Marshall, & Cowley
1995, ISBN 0-8385-9813-7, A9813-5
Clinical Anesthesiology, 2/e
Morgan & Mikhail
1996, ISBN 0-8385-1381-6, A1381-1
Dermatology
Orkin, Maibach, & Dahl
1991, ISBN 0-8385-1288-7, A1288-8
Rudolph's Fundamentals of Pediatrics
Rudolph & Kamei
1994, ISBN 0-8385-8233-8, A8233-7
Genetics in Clinical Medicine and Primary Care
Seashore
1995, ISBN 0-8385-3128-8, A3128-4
Smith's General Urology, 14/e
Tanagho & McAninch
1995, ISBN 0-8385-8612-0, A8612-2
Clinical Oncology
Weiss
1993, ISBN 0-8385-1325-5, A1325-8
General Ophthalmology, 14/e
Vaughan, Asbury, & Riordan-Eva
1995, ISBN 0-8385-3127-X, A3127-6
CURRENT Critical Care Diagnosis &

CURRENT Clinical References

Treatment,
Bongard & Sue
1994, ISBN 0-8385-1443-X, A1443-9
CURRENT Diagnosis & Treatment in Cardiology
Crawford
1995, ISBN 0-8385-1444-8, A1444-7

CURRENT Diagnosis & Treatment in Vascular Surgery
Dean, Yao, & Brewster
1995, ISBN 0-8385-1351-4, A1351-4
CURRENT Obstetric & Gynecologic Diagnosis & Treatment, 8/e
DeCherney & Pernoll
1994, ISBN 0-8385-1447-2, A1447-0
CURRENT Diagnosis & Treatment in Gastroenterology
Grendell, McQuaid, & Friedman
1996, ISBN 0-8385-1448-0, A1448-8
CURRENT Pediatric Diagnosis & Treatment, 12/e
Hay, Groothuis, Hayward, & Levin
1995, ISBN 0-8385-1446-4, A1446-2
CURRENT Emergency Diagnosis & Treatment, 4/e
Saunders & Ho
1993, ISBN 0-8385-1347-6, A1347-2
CURRENT Diagnosis & Treatment in Orthopedics
Skinner
1995, ISBN 0-8385-1009-4, A1009-8
CURRENT Medical Diagnosis & Treatment 1996
Tierney, McPhee, & Papadakis
1996, ISBN 0-8385-1465-0, A1465-2
CURRENT Surgical Diagnosis & Treatment, 10/e
Way
1994, ISBN 0-8385-1439-1, A1439-7

LANGE Clinical Manuals

Dermatology
Diagnosis and Therapy
Bondi, Jegasothy, & Lazarus
1991, ISBN 0-8385-1274-7, A1274-8
Practical Oncology
Cameron
1994, ISBN 0-8385-1326-3, A1326-6
Office & Bedside Procedures
Chesnutt, Dewar, Locksley, & Tureen
1993, ISBN 0-8385-1095-7, A1095-7
Psychiatry
Diagnosis & Therapy 2/e
Flaherty, Davis, & Janicak
1993, ISBN 0-8385-1267-4, A1267-2
Neonatology
Management, Procedures, On-Call Problems, Diseases and Drugs, 3/e
Gomella
1994, ISBN 0-8385-1331-X, A1331-6
Practical Gynecology
Jacobs & Gast
1994, ISBN 0-8385-1336-0, A1336-5
Drug Therapy, 2/e
Katzung
1991, ISBN 0-8385-1312-3, A1312-6

Ambulatory Medicine
The Primary Care of Families
Mengel & Schwiebert
1993, ISBN 0-8385-1294-1, A1294-6
Poisoning & Drug Overdose, 2/e
Olson
1994, ISBN 0-8385-1108-2, A1108-8
Internal Medicine
Diagnosis and Therapy, 3/e
Stein
1993, ISBN 0-8385-1112-0, A1112-0
Surgery
Diagnosis & Therapy
Stillman
1989, ISBN 0-8385-1283-6, A1283-9
Medical Perioperative Management
Wolfsthal
1989, ISBN 0-8385-1298-4, A1298-7

LANGE Handbooks

Handbook of Gynecology & Obstetrics
Brown & Crombleholme
1993, ISBN 0-8385-3608-5, A3608-5
HIV/AIDS Primary Care Handbook
Carmichael, Carmichael, & Fischl
1995, ISBN 0-8385-3557-7, A3557-4
Pocket Guide to Diagnostic Tests
Detmer, McPhee, Nicoll, & Chou
1992, ISBN 0-8385-8020-3, A8020-8
Handbook of Poisoning
Prevention, Diagnosis & Treatment, 12/e
Dreisbach & Robertson
1987, ISBN 0-8385-3643-3, A3643-2
Handbook of Clinical Endocrinology, 2/e
Fitzgerald
1992, ISBN 0-8385-3615-8, A3615-0
Clinician's Pocket Reference, 7/e
Gomella
1993, ISBN 0-8385-1222-4, A1222-7
Surgery on Call, 2/e
Gomella & Lefor
1996, ISBN 0-8385-8746-1, A8746-8
Internal Medicine On Call
Haist & Robbins
1991, ISBN 0-8385-4052-X, A4052-5
Obstetrics & Gynecology On Call
Horowitz & Gomella
1993, ISBN 0-8385-7174-3, A7174-4
Pocket Guide to Commonly Prescribed Drugs
Levine
1993, ISBN 0-8385-8023-8, A8023-2
Handbook of Pediatrics, 17/e
Merenstein, Kaplan, & Rosenberg
1994, ISBN 0-8385-3657-3, A3657-2

 Appleton & Lange • P.O. Box 120041 • Stamford, CT • 06912-0041 • 1-800-423-1359